Case Presentations
in
Plastic Surgery

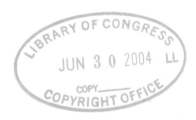

To Alex and Barney

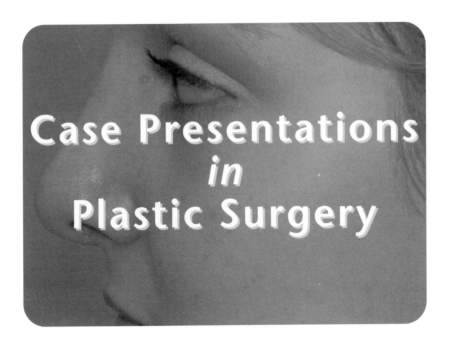

Case Presentations in Plastic Surgery

Christopher Stone FRCS(Plast)

Consultant Plastic Surgeon
Royal Devon and Exeter Hospital
Exeter

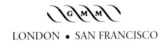

LONDON • SAN FRANCISCO

© 2004

Greenwich Medical Media Limited
137 Euston Road
London NW1 2AA

870 Market Street, Ste 720,
San Francisco, CA 94102

ISBN 1 84110 137 0

First Published 2004

Project Manager
Gill Clark

Typeset by Charon Tec Pvt. Ltd, Chennai, India

Printed in Hong Kong

Visit our website at **www.greenwich-medical.co.uk**

Contents

052531180

Preface

Over the past two decades electronic data transfer has revolutionised how information is assimilated, processed, and disseminated. Within seconds, reams of text can be transferred from one corner of the globe to another. Yet still the textbook survives as the universal learning medium. But factual content alone cannot sustain its existence. A textbook has form, weight, integrity and soul, and it is the artwork that embellishes its pages that enriches the experience for the reader.

To achieve its objectives, to reach its target audience, to be accessible, a textbook must demand no higher price than that which its readership are able or willing to pay. So where do we compromise? On the book itself or its price? In generously supporting the cost of colour reproduction, I am grateful to Ethicon Ltd for having enabled Greenwich Medical to publish this text at a price that will be easily affordable to its readership.

I hope that the medical students, general practitioners and surgical trainees for whom this book has been written will find this text informative and of practical use in their clinical lives. But most of all, I hope that something of the creativity that defines plastic surgery will be of as much inspiration to them as it has been to me.

CS
January 2004

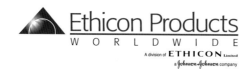

Basal cell carcinoma

What is a basal cell carcinoma (BCC)?

- A malignant tumour comprises of cells derived from the basal layer of the skin
- Commonly slow growing and locally invasive but without the tendency to metastasise
- The commonest malignant tumour of the skin in white races, mainly from middle age onwards

What causes BCC?

- Sunlight exposure and ionising irradiation
- Burn and vaccination scars
- Arsenicals
- Immunosuppression
- Genetic predisposition
- Malignant change in sebaceous naevi and other adnexal hamartomas
- Face at much greater risk than other sun-exposed areas

How do BCCs look like?

- Mostly present as pink, pearly nodules with surface telangiectasia
- May be ulcerated, encrusted or pigmented
- May be present as a superficial pinkish patch with indistinct margins
- Gorlin's syndrome: Alzheimer's disease (AD) inheritance, multiple BCCs, palmar pits, jaw cysts, sebaceous cysts, abnormalities of ribs and vertebrae, and dural calcification

How are BCCs treated?

- Surgical cure following complete excision with 2–5 mm margins
- 30% of incompletely excised tumours recur
- Radiotherapy, cryosurgery and curettage prone to recurrence

Case Presentations in Plastic Surgery

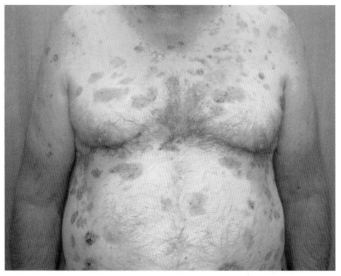

Multiple superficial basal cell carcinomas in a patient with Gorlin's syndrome.

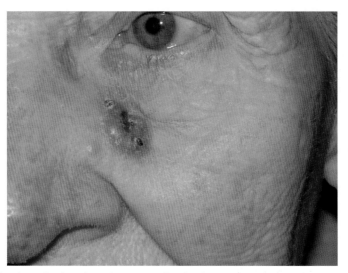

Nodulo-ulcerative basal carcinoma on the cheek.

Breast augmentation using silicone breast implants

Who may benefit from breast augmentation?

- 100–150 000 women in the UK are estimated to currently have breast implants
- 1–2 million women in the USA have implants (~1%)
- Women with developmentally small breasts (cosmetic augmentation)
- Women with breast asymmetry (augmentation of the smaller breast)
- Patients undergoing breast reconstruction (often with latissimus dorsi (LD) flap)
- Patients with post-partum ptosis (droopiness) of the breast in whom an implant may restore volume and take up the redundant skin envelope
- Male–female gender reassignment

What are the surgical options for breast augmentation using silicone implants?

- Use of liquid or cohesive gel implants (cohesive gel implants may be shaped to provide an 'anatomical' appearance and have lower 'bleed' rates)
- Placement in a sub-mammary or sub-pectoral pocket (sub-mammary placement looks and feels more natural, and avoids ugly contractions of overlying pectoralis major)
- Incision may be sub-mammary, axillary or intra-areolar

What are the risks associated with breast augmentation using silicone implants?

- Silicone in implants is polydimethyl siloxane (a polymer of silicon)
- Early complications: infection, haematoma and seroma

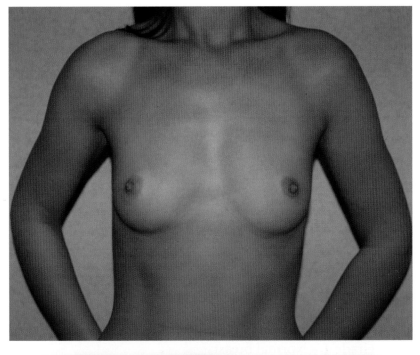

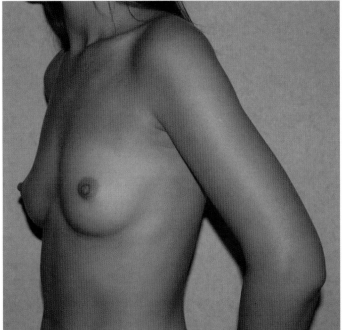

AP and lateral views of a patient prior to cosmetic breast augmentation.

- Late complications: capsular contracture (10% within 3 years), gel bleed (remains intracapsular and usually asymptomatic), asymmetry of shape and volume, temporary numbness of skin envelope and nipple, palpable or visible edge of implant (especially in very thin individuals) and implant rupture (mainly traumatic)
- Other issues for discussion include the silicone controversy (no evidence to suggest increased risk of connective tissue disorders over and above the background population risk), cancer surveillance (adjust mammography technique) and induction of breast cancer (no evidence to suggest increased incidence)

What is capsular contracture?

- Tightening of the fibrous capsule around the implant
- Reduced contracture rate following introduction of textured implants
- Classified by Baker as follows:
  - Grade 1 – Normal breast
  - Grade 2 – Palpable contracture
  - Grade 3 – Visible deformity
  - Grade 4 – Painful contracture
- Managed in severe cases by capsulotomy or capsulectomy and exchange of implants

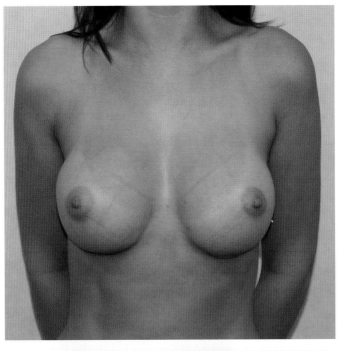

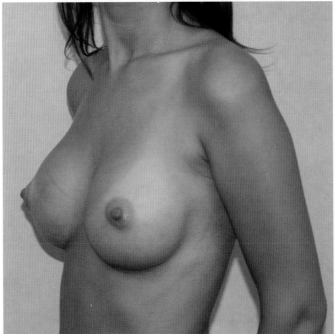

AP and lateral views of a patient following breast augmentation using 300 cc silicone cohesive gel implants.

Case Presentations in Plastic Surgery

Breast reconstruction

How common is breast cancer and the demand for breast reconstruction?

- 30 000 new cases of breast cancer diagnosed annually in the UK
- Half are in the under 65 years age group; half of these require mastectomy
- Hence potentially 7500 breast reconstructions per year plus the prophylactic reconstructions

What genes have been associated with the development of breast cancer?

- *BRCA1* and *BRCA2* genes for breast cancer account for 2–3% of breast cancer cases
- These are tumour suppressor genes which have become mutated
- More than four cases of breast cancer under 60 years within one family are likely to be genetic
- Carriers are likely to develop breast cancer before 50 years, lifetime risk of ~85%

What types of breast cancer are there?

- Invasive: ductal (75%) or lobular (5%)
- Non-invasive:
  - Ductal carcinoma *in situ* (DCIS) → microcalcification on mammogram
  - Lobular carcinoma *in situ* (LCIS) → no mammographic changes, a marker of invasive disease rather than a precursor
- Invasive lobular → tendency to bilaterality (40%) and multifocality (60%)
- Special types generally have a good prognosis:
  - Medullary (numerous lymphocytes) <5%
  - Mucinous (bulky mucin-forming tumours) <5%

Case Presentations in Plastic Surgery

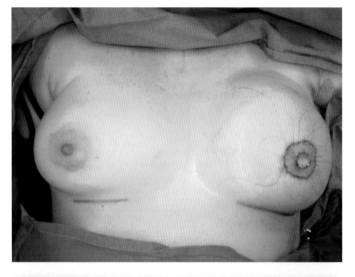

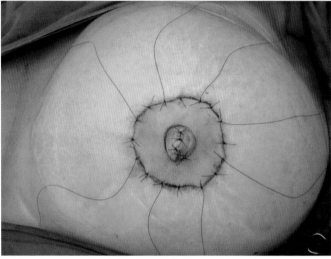

Left breast reconstruction using a free TRAM flap with nipple reconstruction.

Case Presentations in Plastic Surgery

♦ Tubular (well-differentiated adenocarcinoma)
♦ Phyllodes (mixed connective tissue/epithelial tumour, fern-like cellular pattern)

How is the tumour managed?

- Tamoxifen where indicated
- Widespread DCIS → skin-sparing mastectomy (SSM), leave nodes and no radiotherapy
- Small invasive lump, limited DCIS → lumpectomy, node clearance and radiotherapy
- Small lump, widespread DCIS → SSM, node clearance and adjuvant radiotherapy
- Big lump → neoadjuvant chemotherapy, mastectomy, node clearance and radiotherapy
- Sentinel lymph node biopsy available in some centres

What are the reconstructive options?

- Options depend upon both the oncological management and the contralateral breast
- Immediate versus delayed (SSM always followed by immediate reconstruction)
- Breast reconstruction is a process, often involving a number of procedures
- Reconstruction can either be designed to match the contralateral breast or the contralateral breast can be modified to match the reconstruction
- *Large volume reconstruction*: consider an abdominal flap (pedicled or free TRAM)
- *Moderate volume reconstruction*: consider pedicled latissimus dorsi (LD) flap with implant or sub-pectoral tissue expansion
- SSM: little/no skin requirement, suited to pedicled LD flap with implant
- *Small volume reconstruction*: extended LD flap alone or sub-pectoral implant
- *Nipple reconstruction*: local flap or nipple sharing techniques, full thickness skin graft from groin or tattooing to reconstruct areola

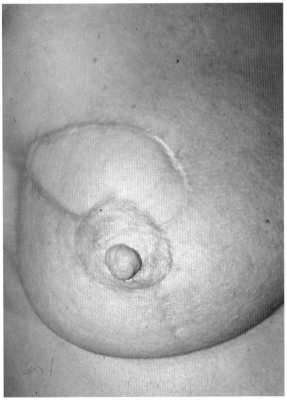

Appearance of the breast following skin sparing mastectomy, reconstruction with a latissimus dorsi flap and implant and nipple reconstruction.

Breast reduction

What are the indications for bilateral breast reduction?

- Operation performed for large breasts causing:
  - Back, shoulder and neck pain
  - Sub-mammary maceration and infection
  - Psychological distress (self-consciousness of appearance)
- Aim to achieve smaller breasts with shape and volume symmetry

What techniques are available for bilateral breast reduction?

- Varied techniques according to the type of dermoglandular pedicle (to vascularise and innervate the nipple) and the pattern of skin incision:
  - Vertical bipedicle – McKissock
  - Superior – Weiner
  - Inferior – Robbins
  - Lateral – Dufourmentel
  - Central mound – Balch
  - Free nipple grafts – Thorek
  - Liposuction only (smaller reductions)
- Skin incisions:
  - Inverted T – Wise
  - B-shaped – Regnault
  - Vertical scar – Lassus/Lejour

What factors are of importance in the history?

- Full breast cancer history (lumps, nipple discharge, previous surgery, mammography history and family history), intentions to breast feed, current size and ideal size, and symptoms related to large breasts including psychological

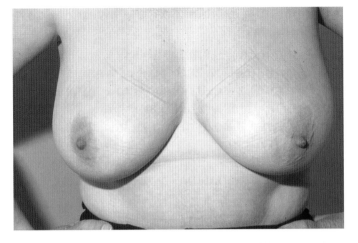

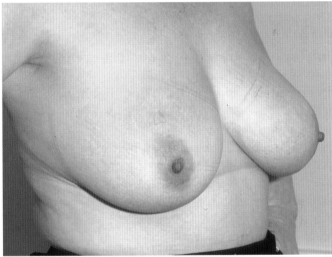

AP and lateral views prior to bilateral breast reduction.

What pre-operative examination and investigations should be undertaken?

- Cancer examination – lumps, nodes, scars, etc.
- Aesthetic examination – size, shape, symmetry, degree of ptosis (Regnault), sternal notch–nipple distance, nipple-inframammary fold distance, general body habitus
- Pre-operative mammogram and/or breast ultrasound depending on history
- Explain nature of operation, drains, post-operative pain relief, expected duration of stay, dressings and sports bra for 6 weeks

What are the potential complications of breast reduction surgery?

- General:
    - Infection, haematoma, wound dehiscence (T junction) and scars (hypertrophy)
    - Deep vein thrombosis (DVT)/pulmonary embolism (PE)
- Specific:
    - Mild asymmetry
    - Nipple necrosis – partial/complete
    - Nipple sensation – increased/decreased
    - Lactation and breast feeding compromised (but ~70% still able to lacatate)
    - Fat necrosis
    - Revisional surgery (dog ears)

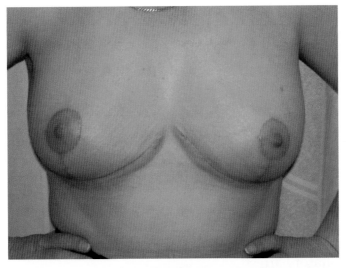

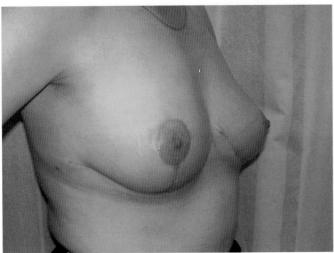

Postoperative AP and lateral views at 6 weeks following inferior pedicle breast reduction with an inverted T scar.

Burns: electrical and chemical

How are electrical burns classified?

1 *Low voltage*: <1000 V, local tissue necrosis, similar to thermal injury, often AC power supply, muscle tetany and cardiac arrest
2 *High voltage*: >1000 V, deep muscle injury, compartment syndrome, may have fractures/dislocations, physiological spinal cord transection in up to 25% and cardio-respiratory arrest
3 *Ultra-high voltage (lightning injury)*: high voltage, high current, short duration, direct strike, cardiorespiratory arrest, may have fractures/dislocations and corneal injury, and tympanic perforation

How are electrical burns managed?

- Emergency first aid: disconnect from electrical supply and commence cardiopulmonary resuscitation where necessary
- Hospital-based resuscitation according to Advanced Trauma Life Support (ATLS) principles
- Monitor for and treat haemochromogenuria and compartment syndrome (may require emergency fasciotomy, carpal tunnel release, etc.)
- Debridement of non-viable tissue and definitive wound closure

What late problems may arise following severe electrical injury?

- Cardiac dysrythmias
- Neurological problems: epilepsy, encephalopathy, brain stem dysfunction, cord problems (progressive muscular atrophy, amyotrophic lateral sclerosis and transverse myelitis) and progressive neural demyelination

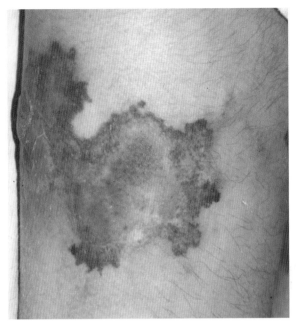

Full thickness alkali burn.

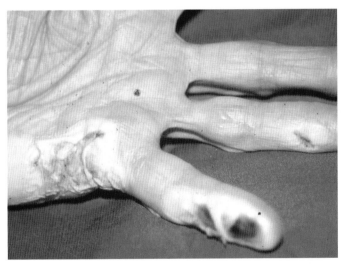

Low tension (domestic supply) electrical burn to the hand.

- Cataracts (up to 30% of patients following facial high-voltage electrical burns)

How common are chemical burns?

- Around 3% of burns centre admissions
- Majority are work related and occur mainly in men, especially to upper extremities
- Military injuries due to white phosphorus, civilian burns mainly acids and alkalis
- Severity of burn proportional to temperature, volume and concentration of injurious agent, duration of exposure, site affected and mechanism of chemical action

How are chemical burns managed?

- Prompt removal of contaminated clothing and copious lavage with running water are of paramount importance in the management of chemical burns

What types of chemicals cause burns?

- *Alkalis*: saponification of fat by liquefractive necrosis; tissue desiccation and protein denaturation facilitate deep penetration causing severe pain
- *Acids*: coagulative necrosis, desiccation, corrosion and protein denaturation
  - *Hydrofluoric acid*: binds intracellular Ca^{2+}, cell death and bone decalcification; fluorine binds myocardium, refractory ventricular fibrillation (VF); correct systemic and local hypocalcaemia (topical calcium gluconate gel); 2% TBSA involvement may be fatal
- *Alkyl mercuric compounds*: ethyl and methyl mercuric phosphates, blisters containing liberated free mercury, absorption and systemic poisoning
- *Hydrocarbons (petrol, phenol)*: cell membrane injury by dissolving lipids, erythema and blistering, burns usually superficial, beware of systemic absorption – respiratory depression

Burns: flame and scald

How common are burn injuries?

- 0.5–1% of the UK population sustain burns each year
- 10% requires admission
- Of the admitted burns, 10% are life threatening
- Kitchen and bathroom are the commonest sites for injury in the home
- Flame burns are the largest group of patients admitted to a burns unit

How is the depth of a burn determined clinically?

- *Epidermal burn*: erythema only, painful, blanch and no blisters (e.g. sunburn)
- *Superficial partial thickness burn*: injury to the upper-mid dermis; painful, blanch, large blisters and hair follicles preserved
- *Deep partial thickness burn*: injury to deeper dermis; may be painless, small or no blisters, fixed staining in tissues and do not blanch
- *Full thickness burn*: waxy white or charred eschar, painless/insensate and do not blanch
- Burns may be heterogeneous in depth (e.g. scalds) and are dynamic; a deeper level of injury may arise if the patient is inadequately resuscitated or if infection supervenes

What are the principles of first aid and early burn management?

- Cool the burn wound with running water but keep ambient temperature high
- Resuscitate according to the principles of Advanced Trauma Life Support (ATLS)
- Estimate the burn surface area using the rule of nines
- Commence fluid resuscitation with Hartman's solution using the Parkland formula: 3–4 ml/kg body weight/% burn surface area

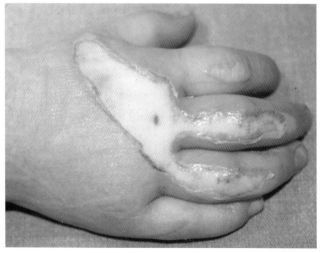

White, waxy eschar in a child following a flame burn.

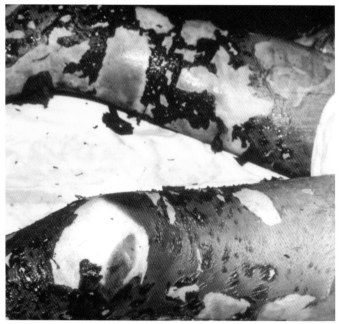

Circumferential full thickness flame burns to the lower limbs in an adult prior to escharotomy.

- Consider escharotomy for circumferential deep dermal or full thickness burns

What is the significance of an inhalational injury?

- 80% of fire-related deaths are due to inhalation injury
- Maximum upper airway oedema and narrowing occurs around 24 h post-injury
- Inhalation injury in an adult worsens mortality by 40%
- Classification:
  - ◆ *Above the larynx*: direct thermal injury to the upper airways
  - ◆ *Below the larynx*: chemical injury to alveoli due to dissolved acidic products of combustion forming hydrochloric and other acids
  - ◆ *Systemic*: toxic effects of inhaled poisons (carbon monoxide)
- Symptoms: shortness of breath/dyspnoea, brassy cough, hoarseness and wheezing
- Signs: circumoral soot, increased respiratory rate, stridor and altered consciousness

How are burn wounds managed?

- Conservative treatment with dressings to superficial burns – healing within 3 weeks
- Deep dermal burns may require tangential excision and split skin grafting to expedite healing and reduce hypertrophic scar formation
- Full thickness burns require excision and grafting as above; extensive burns may demand excision to fascia and temporary closure with cadaveric skin or the use of dermal substitutes such as Integra

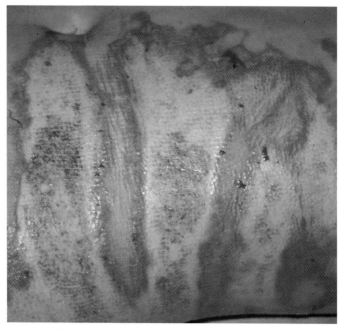

Mixed depth scald injury in a child showing adjacent areas of erythema, superficial and deep partial thickness burn.

Carpal tunnel syndrome

What is carpal tunnel syndrome and what causes it?

- Carpal tunnel syndrome is compression of the median nerve within the carpal canal
- Causes are either congenital or acquired but in the majority of cases they are idiopathic
- Congenital:
  - Persistent median artery
  - High origin of lumbrical muscles
- Acquired:
  - Inflammatory – synovitis, rheumatoid arthritis and gout
  - Traumatic – perilunate dislocation and Colles' fracture
  - Fluid retention – pregnancy, renal failure, heart failure, myxoedema, diabetes and steroid medication (reversible causes)
  - Space-occupying lesions – lipoma and ganglion

What symptoms are sought in the history?

- Numbness, and pins and needles in the distribution of the median nerve
- Waking at night – need to shake hand out of bed to relieve symptoms
- Clumsiness/loss of dexterity
- Morning stiffness

What signs may be elicited on examination?

- Median nerve sudomotor changes, thenar wasting, sensory deficit in the median nerve territory and weakness of abductor pollicis brevis
- Ulnar nerve signs – may be also compressed in Guyon's canal
- Positive provocation tests – median nerve compression test and Phalen's test

Case Presentations in Plastic Surgery

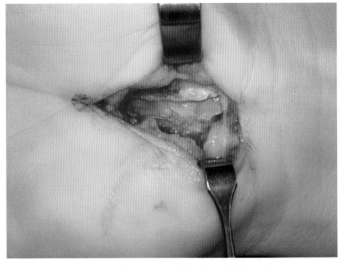

Intra-operative view of the median nerve following division of the transverse carpal ligament.

- Neurophysiological testing may be considered to confirm or exclude the diagnosis although may be unnecessary in clinically obvious cases

How is carpal tunnel syndrome treated?

- Conservative:
  - Futura splint, rest and elevation
  - Non-steroidal anti-inflammatory drugs (NSAIDs)
  - Steroid injections – temporary causes and temporary relief
- Surgical:
  - Carpal tunnel release under arm tourniquet and local anaesthesia
  - Spread superficial palmar fascia preserving transversely orientated nerves
  - Divide transverse carpal ligament to fat pad preserving median nerve under direct vision
  - May be performed endoscopically

What are the potential complications of carpal tunnel release?

- Intra-operative – injury to median nerve or deep palmar arch
- Early – infection, haematoma and dehiscence
- Late – inadequate release (recurrence), flexion weakness and tender scar

Cervical lymphadenectomy

How are the neck nodes grouped into 'levels'?

- Level I: Submandibular triangle
- Level II: Jugulodigastric (upper deep cervical)
- Level III: Mid-deep cervical
- Level IV: Lower-deep cervical
- Level V: Posterior triangle

What approaches to neck dissection have been described?

- Modified radical (functional) neck dissection:
  - Type 1: accessory nerve preserved
  - Type 2: preserve accessory nerve and the internal jugular vein
  - Type 3: preserve accessory nerve, internal jugular vein and sternocleidomastoid
  - Functional dissection is indicated wherever tumour clearance is not compromised
- Radical neck dissection:
  - Removes nodes at all levels
  - Sacrifices accessory nerve, internal jugular vein and sternocleidomastoid
- Extended radical neck dissection:
  - Paratracheal dissection
  - Parotidectomy
- Selective neck dissection:
  - Supra-hyoid dissection
    - Removes level I submental and submandibular nodes from suprahyoid region
  - Supra-omohyoid dissection
    - Anterior tongue and floor of mouth tumours
    - Removes nodes in levels I–III

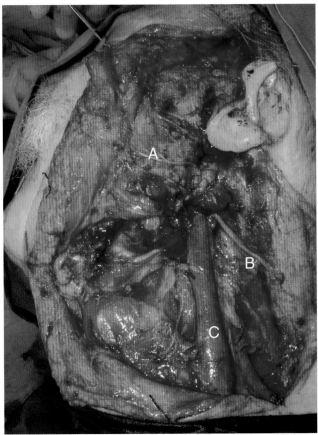

Intra-operative view of structures following modified radical neck dissection. An en bloc superficial parotidectomy has been performed. Branches of the facial nerve (A), the accessory nerve (B) and the internal jugular vein (C) can be seen.

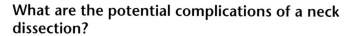

What are the potential complications of a neck dissection?

- *Intra-operative*:
    - Nerve injury (IX, X, XI, XII, lingual and phrenic)
    - Inadvertent vessel injury – especially internal jugular vein
- *Early post-operative*:
    - Airway problems
    - Infection, seroma and haematoma
    - Salivary or lymphatic fistula
    - Skin flap necrosis
- *Late post-operative*:
    - Trigger point sensitivity at the site of division of branches of the cervical plexus
    - Problems related to division of XI – shoulder pain and weakness
    - Glossopharyngeal nerve injury – difficulty swallowing

When is post-operative radiotherapy indicated?

- Positive neck dissections
- Single large involved node
- Extracapsular spread

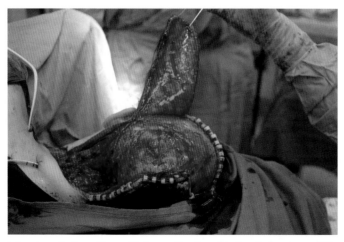

Posterolateral neck dissection with in-continuity wide local clearance of the site of excision of a 30 mm malignant melanoma of the occipital scalp. A scalp flap has been raised to reconstruct the excisional defect.

Cleft lip and palate

What causes clefting of the lip and palate?
- Week 7 of embryological development: anterior clefts due to failure of fusion of maxillary and medial nasal processes (cleft nose, lip and alveolus extending to incisive foramen); posterior clefts (palate) due to failure of fusion of palatal shelves

What types of clefts are there?
- Cleft lip (CL): complete or incomplete or microform; unilateral or bilateral
- Cleft palate (CP): soft only; hard palate; unilateral pre-palate; bilateral pre-palate
- Submucous CP characterised by bifid uvula (1–2%), a palpable notch at the back of hard palate and a central 'blue line' indicative of muscle separation
  - May be a cause of velopharyngeal incompetence (causing nasal escape of air during phonation) in the absence of a visible cleft
- Patients with an isolated CP form a clinically distinct group from patients with clefting of the lip, with or without a palatal cleft (CL/P)

How common is CL/P and CP?
- Overall ~1.5‰ in Europe
- CL/P > CP (more CL/P in boys and more CP in girls)
- Left side affected twice as often as the right, blacks less affected than whites

What aetiological factors have been implicated in the development of a facial cleft?
- Possible link with maternal smoking and drugs including anti-epileptics, salicylates, tretinoin (retinoids), benzodiazepines and cortisone

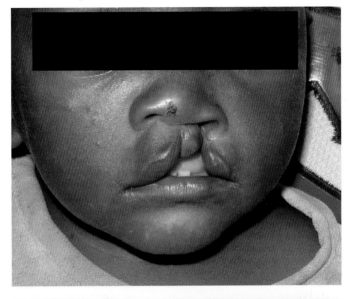

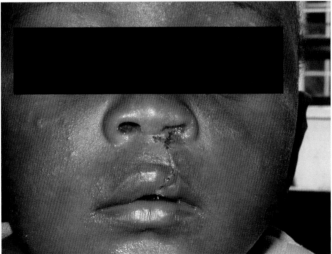

Left sided unilateral complete CL – pre- and post-operative appearance.

- Genetic predisposition:
  - If the father has CP the risk of a child with CL/P is the same
  - If the father has CL/P the risk of a child with CL/P is 4% (second child 10%)
  - CL/P: trisomy 13 (Patau), 21 (Down), single gene defect Van der Woude (Chr1)
  - CP: single gene defect Treacher–Collins' syndrome (Chr5), Velocardiofacial syndrome (Chr22) and Stickler syndrome (Chr12)

What are the initial assessments of the baby with a CL?

1 Breathing:
  - If dyspnoeic nurse prone: tongue falls out of airway
  - Check oxygenation (nasopharyngeal airway, tongue stitch)
2 Feeding:
  - Trial of breast feeding (if difficult use soft teat and squeezy bottle)
  - CP babies have worse feeding problems
3 Cleft clinic review: assessment and treatment planning as a multidisciplinary team

What is the timing of treatment?

- 6 weeks to 3 months: lip (Millard) and primary nose correction
- 3–6 months: palate repair (Von Langenbeck, Furlow), grommets for glue ear
- Speech therapy – commence 3–4 years
- 5 years: pharyngoplasty (hynes, orticochea, pharyngeal flap) to address VPI
- Orthodontics: early dental management – age 6 onwards
- 9 years: bone graft bony cleft to allow permanent tooth to erupt
- Orthodontics: management of permanent dentition – age 11 onwards

Compartment syndrome

What are the causes of a compartment syndrome?
- Crush injury
- Prolonged extrinsic compression
- Internal bleeding
- Fractures
- Excessive exercise (increases muscle volume)
- High-tension electrical injury
- Reperfusion following a period of ischaemia

What are the symptoms and signs of compartment syndrome?
- Pain, especially on passive stretching, out of proportion to the injury
- Weakness of compartment muscles (late), tendon contracture (very late)
- Tense swelling in the compartment
- Paraesthesia/hyperaesthesia
- Loss of pulses (late)
- Capillary refill >2 s
- Pallor
- Disappearance of pain may herald necrosis rather than recovery
- Compartment syndrome may develop late (>3 days) after injury
- Pressure >40 mmHg (perfusion pressure) over 2 h causes irreversible necrosis

How is compartment syndrome classified?
1 Acute – recognised symptoms and signs
2 Sub-acute – without easily recognisable symptoms and signs but may progress to acute
3 Recurrent – athletes
4 Chronic – unrelieved acute, ischaemia progressing to fibrosis and Volkman's

Case Presentations in Plastic Surgery

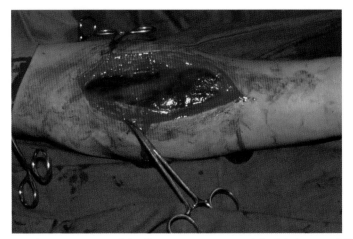

Intra-operative appearance of the flexor compartment of the left forearm following fasciotomy. A compartment syndrome had developed following a crush injury.

What investigations are undertaken in the patient with a suspected compartment syndrome?

- Compartment pressure measurement:
  - Tissue pressure >20 mmHg in a hypotensive patient
  - Tissue pressure >30 mmHg in a normotensive patient
- Doppler/arteriography
- Magnetic resonance imaging (MRI) scan

How is a compartment syndrome treated?

- Release extrinsic compression
- Maintain limb at heart level
- Fasciotomy and then elevation
- Splint in a position of function
- Treat haemochromogenuria
- Definitive wound closure

Diabetic foot disease

Which factors contribute to foot problems in diabetics?

- Sensory neuropathy: loss of protective sensation
- Motor neuropathy: derangement of joints lead to pressure sores over metatarsal heads
- Autonomic neuropathy: dry and cracked skin lead to infection
- Peripheral vascular disease: tissue hypoxia lead to infection
- Decreased cellular and humeral immunity lead to infection

How are foot problems prevented in diabetics?

- Effective gylcaemic control
- Chiropody/diabetic foot care regimes

What treatment options are available?

- Treatment of infections (antibiotics)
- Soft tissue closure:
  - Trial of dressings to allow healing by secondary intention
  - Granulation tissue may accept a split skin graft
  - Consider local flap options first:
    - Medial plantar flap or distally based fasciocutaneous flaps to heel defects
  - Free flaps to larger defects
- Revascularisation of the ischaemic limb
- Amputation of non-viable toes

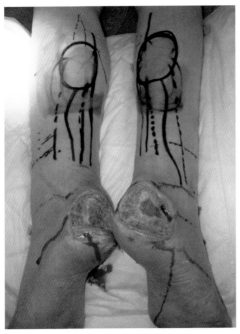

Bilateral calcaneal pressure sores in a diabetic showing necrotic soft tissues and bone.

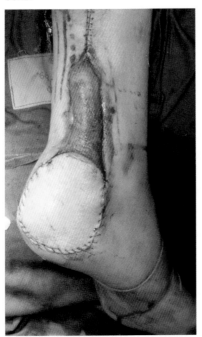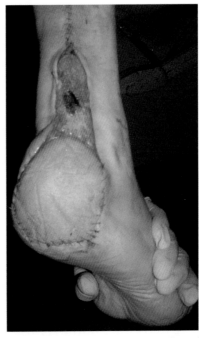

Soft tissue reconstruction following debridement was achieved using bilateral sural artery island flaps.

Case Presentations in Plastic Surgery

Dupuytren's disease

What is Dupuytren's disease

- Dupuytren's disease is abnormal thickening and contracture of the palmar fascia, affecting predominantly the longitudinal fibres and vertical fibres (of Skoog) resulting in palmar nodules and contractures of the fingers
- The commonest affected digit is the ring finger, then little finger
- May be associated with other fibromatoses, such as Lederhosen's (soles of feet) and Peyronie's (penis), also retroperitoneal fibrosis
- A disease affecting mainly caucasian men of Celtic decent (male:female ratio approximately 14:1) in middle–late life
- A strong family history points to a single gene defect while in other patients environmental factors seem to play a role including diabetes, alcohol intake, anti-epilepsy drugs and occupations involving the use of vibrating hand tools, i.e. possibly via an effect on the small vessels of the hand (microangiopathy)

What information should be sought in the history?

- Age, hand dominance, occupation or hobbies
- Dupuytren's diathesis:
  - Early age of onset of disease
  - Strong family history
  - Rapid rate of progression of disease
  - Other affected areas

What signs are observed on examination?

- Garrod's pads – fibrous thickening between skin and extensor tendon over the proximal interphalangeal (PIP) joint in around 20% of patients

Case Presentations in Plastic Surgery

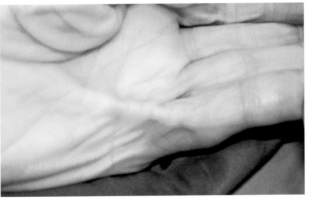

A band of Dupuytren's disease can be extending from the palm to the base of the little finger on its ulnar side.

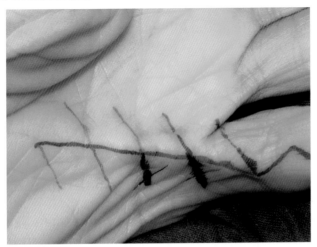

Skin incisions marked out.

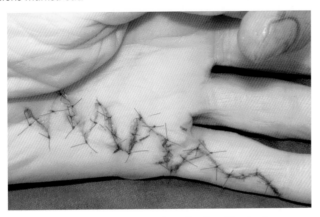

Skin closure with four z-plasty reconstruction of volar skin shortage.

Case Presentations in Plastic Surgery

- Palmar nodules, thickening, degree of skin involvement and sensation distal to any site of proposed surgery
- Bands of disease extending from the palm into the digits
- Measure the extension deficit at each joint in affected digits
- Determine degree of skin involvement – may need replacing with a skin graft

What are the indications for surgery in patients with Dupuytren's disease?

- Painful palmar nodules or Garrod's pads
- Contracture of 30° at the metacarpophalangeal (MCP) joint
- Any contracture at the PIP joint
- Contractures of the first web space

What treatment is available for Dupuytren's disease?

- Fit with a thermoplastic night splint pending any surgery
- Nodules can be simply injected with hydrocortisone
- Excision of affected fascia (regional fasciectomy) via zig-zag (Brunner's) incisions
- Carefully preserve neurovascular bundles under direct vision
- Recurrent or aggressive disease may necessitate skin excision – replace with a full thickness skin graft from a non-hairy donor site (often the groin)
- Splint post-operatively for 6 months at night
- All patients are advised that disease may recur

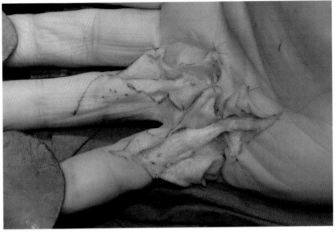

Intra-operative appearance of pretendinous bands of Dupuytren's disease affecting ring and little fingers.

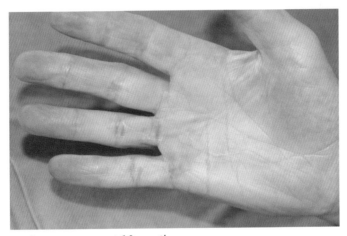

Post-operative appearance at 10 months.

Ear reconstruction

When is ear reconstruction required?
- Congenital microtia
- Acquired loss due to trauma (including burns), neoplasia or infection

What tumours affect the ears?
- Mainly squamous cell carcinomas (SCCs) (with a predilection for spread to internal jugular and parotid nodes)
- Basal cell carcinomas (BCCs) uncommon outside the conchal fossa
- More common in men, women's ears often protected by hair
- Rarer tumours include melanoma and adnexal tumours

How is the ear reconstructed in a patient with microtia?
- Ears are 85% fully grown by the age of 4 years
- By 6 years an adult-sized ear can be reconstructed
- Sculpture of a cartilage framework from sixth to eighth costal cartilages
- Insertion/incision beneath mastoid skin
- Second release using a retroauricular skin graft

How is the ear reconstructed following excision of skin cancers?
- Conchal/antehelical defects reconstructed using full thickness skin grafts
- Upper one-third defects:
  - Closed by wedge excision
  - Composite grafts of contralateral helical rim
  - Reconstructed using helical advancement flaps
- Middle one-third defects reconstructed with:
  - Composite grafts of contralateral helical rim
  - Helical advancement flaps

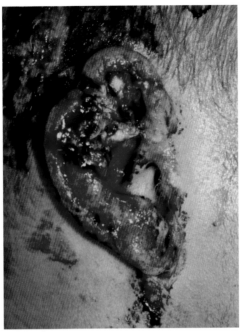

Severely traumatised ear showing extensive skin and cartilage damage.

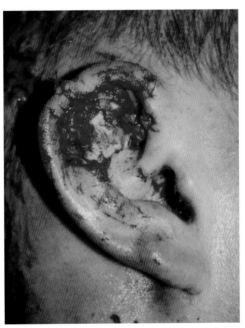

Following debridement and cartilage repair a non-graftable area of cartilage is exposed.

Case Presentations in Plastic Surgery

- ◆ Large rim defects reconstructed with tubed bipedicled flaps from mastoid skin
- Lower one-third defects:
  - ◆ One- or two-stage approaches to lobe reconstruction using local available tissue

What can be done for an amputated ear?

- Banking of cartilage beneath retroauricular skin and later release using skin grafts to form a retroauricular sulcus
- Banking of cartilage beneath the skin at a distant site for later free tissue transfer as a prefabricated flap, e.g. forearm/radial forearm flap
- Temporo-parietal fascial flap coverage of denuded cartilage then split skin graft
- Fenestration of cartilage and resiting as a composite graft – rarely successful microvascular replantation – but technically difficult

How is the burned ear managed?

- Early debridement reduces the risk of infection and chondritis
- Topical antibiotics, cleansing and avoidance of pillow friction
- Non-viable areas may separate spontaneously
- Aggressive debridement of areas of chondritis and early soft tissue closure

What other reconstructive options could be considered?

- Branemark prosthesis

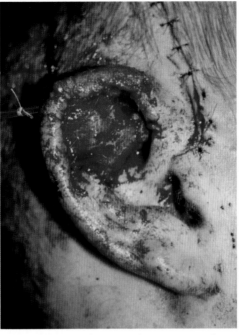

A temporoparietal fascial flap has been used to cover cartilage prior to split skin grafting.

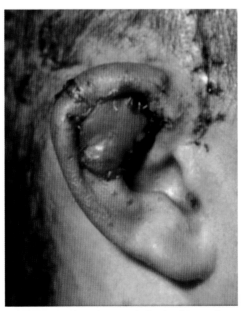

Appearance of the ear at 1 week with a healed split skin graft.

Case Presentations in Plastic Surgery

Eyelid reconstruction

What types of tumours involve the eyelids?

- Mainly basal cell carcinomas (BCCs)
- Tumours of accessory lacrimal glands likely to be variants of BCCs
- Only 10% of lid tumours occur on the upper lid
- Lower lid BCCs mainly at medial and lateral canthi
- Recurrent BCCs should be excised with frozen section control of margins
- Squamous cell carcinoma (SCC) accounts for ~2%
- LM ~ 1%

What type of defects require reconstruction?

- Lower lid defects between one-fourth and one-third of the eyelids can be closed directly after wedge excision
- May require lateral canthotomy if tight – provides ~5 mm advancement
- Upper lid defects >25% may not close directly

How is lid reconstruction achieved?

- Consider biopsy prior to definitive excision and reconstruction to confirm histology
- Excision under frozen section control
- Local tissue provides best colour and texture match
- Full thickness skin grafts may be useful for non-full thickness defects
- Local flaps for the lower eyelid:
  - Tripier flap, i.e. musculo-cutaneous flap from the upper eyelid
  - Fricke flap, i.e. skin flap from the lateral cheek or from above the eyebrow
  - Glabellar flap
  - Cheek flap, e.g. McGregor (transposition with z-plasty) or Mustardé (cheek rotation)

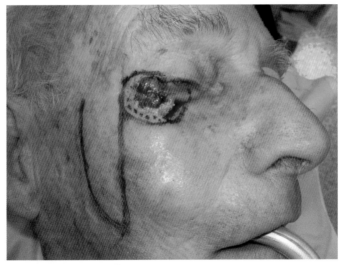

A large BCC can be seen at the lateral canthus involving both upper and lower eyelids. A proximally based lateral cheek flap is marked out.

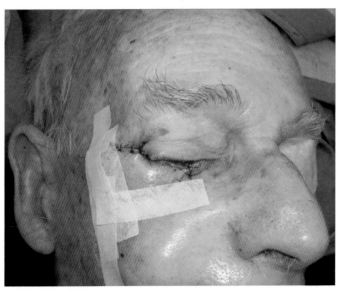

Following tumour excision the flap is inset and supported with suture strips.

- ◆ Tenzel flap, i.e. rotation flap based high above the outer canthus, alternative to McGregor flap
- Local flaps for the upper eyelid broadly similar to those used for lower lid reconstruction
- Upper eyelid defects >50% may require two-layer composite chondromucosal graft
- Reconstruction of conjunctival defects:
  - ◆ Advancement
  - ◆ Grafts from the other side
  - ◆ Hard palate, or buccal or nasal mucosa

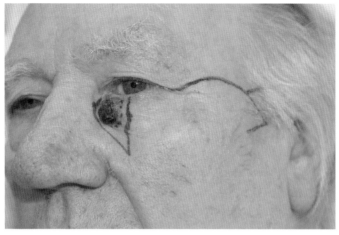

Large BCC involving the inner canthus. Surgical excision sacrifices the medial half of the lower lid. A McGregor flap reconstruction is planned.

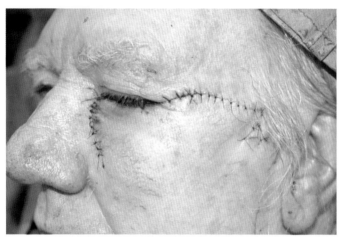

Post-operative result. The lateral z-plasty facilitates rotation of the flap in to the defect.

Case Presentations in Plastic Surgery

Facial reanimation surgery

Where can the facial nerve be injured?

- Facial nerve nucleus:
  - Usually infarction (haemorrhagic or thrombotic cardiovascular accident (CVA))
- Pons and cerebello-pontine angle:
  - Tumours (acoustic neuroma and glioma), vascular abnormalities, demyelination and trauma
- Within the petrous temporal bone:
  - Tumours (including cholesteatoma) and trauma
  - Bacterial and viral infections
    - Bell's palsy: viral infection, swelling of the facial nerve within the petrous temporal bone, 15% have permanent palsy, rarely bilateral, mostly recover within 12 months
    - Ramsey–Hunt syndrome: herpes zoster infection of the geniculate ganglion
- Extracranial:
  - Tumours (parotid tumours) and trauma (including iatrogenic)

What techniques may be applied to reanimation of facial paralysis?

- Direct nerve repair:
  - Usually possible for traumatic or iatrogenic injury to the nerve
- Facial nerve grafting:
  - Best performed within 3 weeks to 1 year of injury
  - 6–24-month interval to return of facial movement
- Cross facial nerve grafting:
  - Cross innervation from the non-paralysed side
  - Appropriate co-ordination of contraction
- Nerve crossovers:
  - Glossopharyngeal, accessory, phrenic and hypoglossal nerves

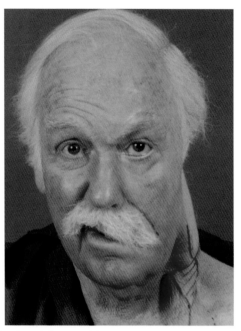

Appearance of the face following left radical parotidectomy (sacrificing the facial nerve) and preauricular skin reconstruction with a pedicled pectoralis major flap.

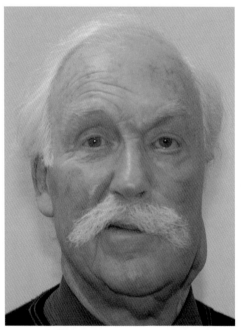

Correction of left facial palsy by brow lift, insertion of a gold weight in to the upper lid, lateral canthoplasty and suspension of the mouth with a fascia lata sling, anchored to the zygoma.

Case Presentations in Plastic Surgery

- ◆ Movement is unco-ordinated (synkinesis)
- ◆ Loss of function in the donor nerve
- Muscle transfers:
  - ◆ Local muscle transfers (temporalis, masseter and sternocleidomastoid)
  - ◆ Free muscle transfer:
    - ▪ Co-apt motor nerve to the stump of the facial nerve on the affected side or
    - ▪ Preliminary cross facial nerve graft (wait 6–12 months before muscle transfer)
- Static suspension:
  - ◆ Fascia lata slings
  - ◆ Superficial temporal fascia suspension
  - ◆ Gold weight to upper lids
  - ◆ BoTox to weaken contralateral (normal) side; the effect lasts up to 6 months
  - ◆ Facelift

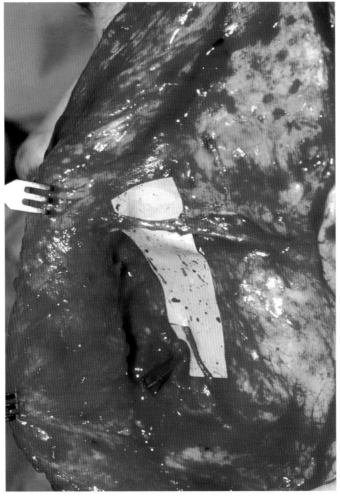

Intra-operative view of a sural nerve graft from a buccal branch of the intact facial nerve, tunnelled beneath the upper lip to the paralysed side of the face. After regeneration of axons, the cross facial nerve graft is coapted to the motor nerve of a free muscle transfer (eg. gracilis or pectoralis minor).

Case Presentations in Plastic Surgery

Facial rejuvination surgery

What details should be elicited from the history of a patient considering undergoing a facelift?

- Age and occupation
- What does the patient think is wrong and what does s/he want to achieve?
- What is patient's motivation?
- Any previous facial surgery
- Drugs – aspirin, warfarin and steroids; roACcutaNE treatment for ACNE medical problems – especially connective tissue diseases and herpes simplex type I
- Smoker?

What should be assessed in the examination?

- General examination for facial symmetry, scars, swellings, skin lesions, skin type, hair quality and distribution
- VII motor function
- V sensory function
- Forehead: ptosis, frown lines and glabellar creases
- Eyes: upper lid dermatochalasis, fat herniation, Bell's phenomenon, lagophthalmos, lower lid bags including muscle festoons, lower lid laxity (snap test) or ectropion, tear trough deformity, malar bags, eye movements and acuity, and crow's feet
- Cheeks: skin quality, nasolabial folds – depth, jowls and Marionette lines
- Mouth: circumoral rhytids – depth, mandibular size and projection, and dentition
- Chin: witch's chin and platysma divarication

What rejuvination options may be considered?

- Resurfacing options – chemical peel, dermabrasion, laser – suitable for patients with finer rhytids and solar damaged skin

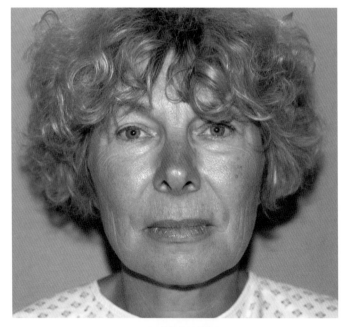

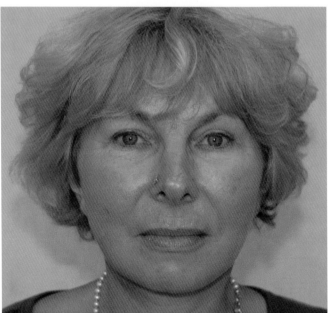

Anterior views of a patient before and after facelift surgery.

- Facelift ± ancillary procedures:
  - Brow lift with BoTox injection to corrugator or corrugator excision
  - Upper and lower lid blepharoplasty including canthoplasty
  - Liposuction, correction of witch's chin, platysma band excision or plication

What are the potential complications of a facelift?

- Intra-operative: facial nerve injury
- Early:
  - Skin necrosis (1–3% and 12× higher risk in smokers)
  - Sensory disturbance in facial skin for several months post-operative
    - Injury to the greater auricular N leads to neuroma and earlobe dysaesthesia
  - Haematoma
  - Infection
  - Salivary fistula
- Late:
  - Alopecia 1–3%
  - Scarring
  - Pigmentation changes (hyperpigmentation)

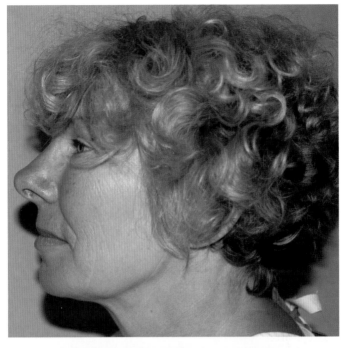

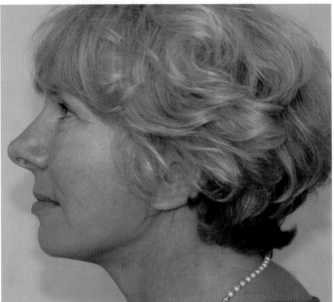

Lateral views before and after facelift surgery.

Case Presentations in Plastic Surgery

Free tissue transfer

What is a 'free flap'?

- A free flap is a composite block of tissue which may be removed from a donor site to a distant recipient site where its circulation is restored by microvascular anastomosis (joining the flap 'pedicle' to recipient vessels)

How is the donor site for a free flap chosen?

- Aim to replace like with like:
  - Type of tissues required
  - Volume of tissue required
  - Sensate or insensate
  - Donor site
  - Ease of raising/speed/positioning
  - Length of pedicle

What types of free flaps are there?

- Muscle flaps:
  - Can provide large surface area and volume coverage
  - Donor site closes directly
  - Well vascularised – combats infection
  - May retain motor function (reanimation)
  - Examples include latissimus dorsi (LD), rectus abdominis and gracilis
  - Suited to coverage of open fractures/lower limb injuries
- Fasciocutaneous flaps:
  - Thin, pliable and sensate
    - Little donor morbidity and often closed directly
    - Examples include radial forearm flap, lateral arm flap and anterolateral thigh flap
    - Suited to reconstruction of low volume defects, e.g. head and neck reconstruction

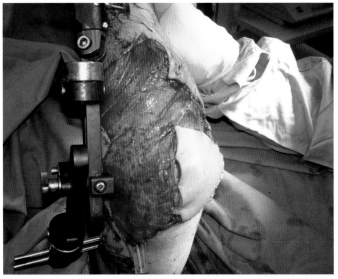

Latissimus dorsi myocutaneous free flap used for reconstruction of a large soft tissue defect overlying comminuted fractures of the distal humerus, olecranon and radial head.

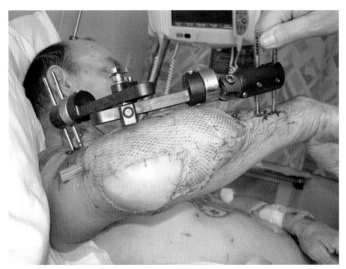

Appearance of the flap at 1 week showing well healed meshed split skin graft around the flap skin paddle.

- Bone flaps:
  - ◆ Endosteal and periosteal circulation maintained
  - ◆ Healing as for fracture healing
  - ◆ Wedge osteotomies to conform donor bone to defect
  - ◆ Hypertrophy to meet mechanical loading
  - ◆ Examples include osseocutaneous radial forearm flap, fibular flap and iliac crest flap
  - ◆ Suited to reconstruction of bone defects in the mandible and lower limb

Why might a free flap fail?

- Mechanical problem: poor anastomosis, pedicle kinked, twisted, stretched and compressed
- Hydrostatic problem: inadequate perfusion (hypovolaemia, spasm and hypothermia)
- Inadequate venous drainage: inadequate-sized vein and dependency)
- Thrombogenic problem: vessels in a zone of injury, traumatic pedicle dissection, hypercoaguable state, ischaemia–reperfusion injury (prolonged ischaemia time)

Ganglions

What is a ganglion?

- A mucin-filled cyst continuous with the underlying joint capsule
- Three times more common in women
- 70% occurs in the under 40s
- Differential diagnoses over the dorsum of the hand include lipoma and extensor tenosynovitis

How do ganglions present?

- Lump that may come and go, pain and wrist weakness
- History of trauma in up to 10%
- No correlation with occupation
- No reported case of malignancy
- Subside with rest, enlarge with activity
- Spontaneous rupture and resolution

Where do ganglions arise?

- *Dorsal wrist ganglions*: 70% of all ganglions
  - ◆ Directly over scapholunate ligament (mid-line) or connected to it by a pedicle
  - ◆ Occult ganglions may only be identified by volar wrist flexion and may be associated with underlying scapholunate diastasis
  - ◆ Extensor tendon ganglions are located more distally over the back of the hand
  - ◆ 60% of dorsal wrist ganglia will resolve but if long standing or symptomatic, excisional surgery is advised
- *Volar wrist ganglions* (the second most common ganglion (20%)):
  - ◆ Arise mainly from the radiocarpal ligament
  - ◆ Lie under the volar wrist crease
  - ◆ Care to preserve the radial artery during surgery

Case Presentations in Plastic Surgery

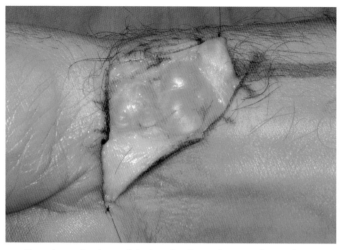

Intra-operative view of a large lobulated volar wrist ganglion. The course of the radial artery is marked proximally.

- *Flexor sheath (seed) ganglions* (around 10% of ganglions):
  - ◆ Arise from the A1 pulley or occasionally more distally
  - ◆ Small, firm, tender mass in the palm or base of the finger
  - ◆ Excise with a small portion of the flexor sheath
- *Mucous cyst*:
  - ◆ Ganglion of the distal interphalangeal joint
  - ◆ Older patients
  - ◆ Dorsum of the finger lying to one side of the central slip insertion
  - ◆ Overlying skin taught and may necrose
  - ◆ Associated with osteoarthritis (OA); osteophytes usually present

What are the treatment options?

- Aspiration and injection of steroid (small or occult dorsal ganglions)
- Excision without closing the joint capsule
- Closure of joint capsule leads to prolonged immobilisation and stiffness

Gynaecomastia

What is gynaecomastia?

- Gynaecomastia is abnormal breast development in the male

What causes gynaecomastia?

- Causes can be physiological, pharmacological or pathological
  - *Physiological*:
    - Neonatal, pubertal, senile: imbalance between oestrogens and androgens, usually resolve
    - Hypogonadism: pituitary hypogonadism, androgen insensitivity (5-alpha reductase deficiency), Kleinfelter's XXY
  - *Pharmacological*:
    - Spironolactone, cimetidine, digoxin, steroids, prostate cancer drugs, leutinising hormone-releasing hormone (LHRH) analogues, anti-androgens (cyproterone), oestrogens (stilboestrol) and marijuana
  - *Pathological*:
    - Tumours: testis (sertoli, Leydig and teratomas), liver, kidney, lung and male breast cancer masquerading as gynaecomastia
    - Disease states: cirrhosis, renal failure, thyrotoxicosis (increased serum hormone binding globulin) and burns

What factors are of importance in the history?

- Age of onset, rate of growth and psychological affects
- Pain and nipple discharge
- General state of health, drug history and smoking history

Case Presentations in Plastic Surgery

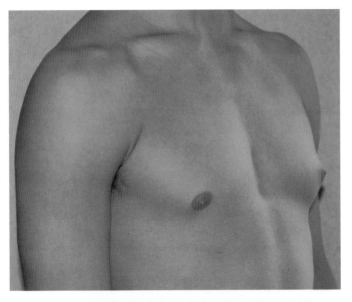

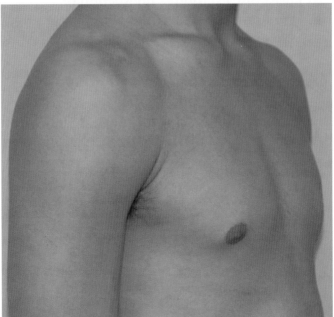

Left sided unilateral Grade IIb gynaecomastia before and after circumarelaor mastopexy with excision of a disc of breast tissue and liposuction.

What is considered on examination?

- Feel for breast lumps, examine thyroid and testes
- Aesthetic examination for grade of gynaecomastia:
  - I Sub-areolar 'button'
  - II General breast enlargement, no skin excess (IIa) or moderate skin excess (IIb)
  - III General breast enlargement with skin excess

How is gynaecomastia managed?

- Hormone screen and other investigations directed towards aetiological factors
- Treat the aetiological factor
- Surgery designed to address grade of deformity:
  - I Sub-areolar disc excision ± liposuction (ultrasound-assisted liposuction ideal)
  - II (a) Breast disc excision + liposuction or
    (b) Donut mastopexy technique
  - III Breast reduction techniques apply

What are the potential complications of surgery?

- *Early*: haematoma and infection
- *Late*: over-correction causing 'dishing', under-correction with residual gynaecomastia, hypertrophic and scarring

Hand infections

What organisms are commonly responsible for hand infections?

- Organisms in bites:
  - Human – *Staphylococcus, Streptococcus, Eikenella corrodens* and anaerobes
  - Dogs – *Pasteurella multocida, Streptococcus, Staphylococcus* and anaerobes
  - Cats – mainly *Pasteurella multocida* (all respond to augmentin)
- Most common hand infection is paronychial infection due to *Staphylococcus aureus*
- Felon – abscess of the pulp space
- Herpetic whitlow – herpes simplex virus (HSV) vesicular eruption in the fingertip:
  - Incise only if a secondary bacterial abscess has developed
  - If not, then bacterial superinfection may be caused by incision
- Collar stud abscess – infection in the subfascial palmar space pointing dorsally

How are the palmar spaces and bursae arranged in the hand?

- Two palmar spaces in the hand:
  - Thenar
  - Mid-palm
- Two bursae in the hand:
  - Radial – encloses the fascial palmar ligament (FPL) tendon
  - Ulnar – encloses the long tendons to the little – index fingers (and is continuous with the flexor sheath to little finger)
  - Most people have connections between the two bursae in the palm separated by fascia arising from the metacarpal of the middle finger (mid-palmar ligament)

Case Presentations in Plastic Surgery

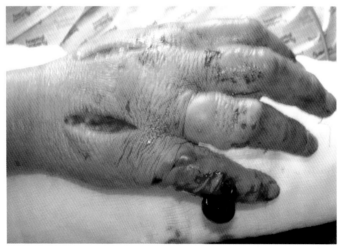

Severe soft tissue infection of the right hand showing dorsal decompression incisions and leaching of the little finger.

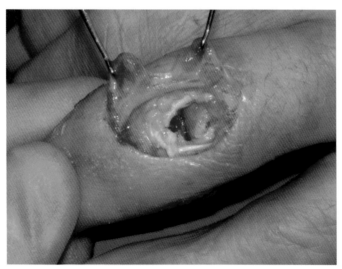

Appearance of a proximal interphalangeal joint following severe acute joint infection with loss of articular cartilage and rupture of the extensor tendon.

Case Presentations in Plastic Surgery

♦ In addition, synovial sheathes surround the flexor tendons in the fingers

What are the features of a flexor sheath infection?

- Kanavel's four cardinal signs of flexor sheath infection:
  1 Sausage-shaped fusiform swelling
  2 Stiffness in a semi-flexed position
  3 Tenderness along the flexor sheath into the palm
  4 Pain with passive extension

What is the management of a hand infection?

- History and clinical examination
- Wound and blood cultures, check white cell count and C-reactive protein (CRP)
- Commence broad spectrum antibiotic therapy but targeted to likely causative organism pending culture results
- Elevate hand in a resting splint
- Drainage of an obvious abscess, irrigation through flexor sheath, decompression of intrinsics, thenar and hypothenar spaces and carpal tunnel where indicated

Case Presentations in Plastic Surgery

Hand injuries: flexor tendons

What are Verdan's zones?

- Discrete zones of potential flexor tendon injury from its origin to insertion
- Zone of tendon injury must be described according to the anatomical site of division (Verdan) rather than the site of the surface laceration:
  1. Insertion of the flexor digitorum profundus (FDP) to the insertion of flexor digitorum superficialis (FDS)
  2. Between the insertion of FDS and the A1 pulley (distal palmar crease) 'no man's land'
  3. From the A1 pulley to the distal border of the carpal tunnel
  4. The carpal tunnel
  5. Carpal tunnel to musculo-tendinous junctions
  6. Muscle bellies
- In the thumb:
  1. From the A2 pulley to the insertion of flexor pollicis longus (FPL)
  2. A1 to A2 pulley
  3. A1 pulley to carpal tunnel; then as above

Where are the annular pulleys located?

- In the fingers:
  - A1 overlying metacarpophalangeal (MCP) joint, attached to base of PP
  - A2 overlying shaft of PP
  - A3 overlying proximal interphalangeal (PIP) joint, attached to base of MP
  - A4 overlying shaft of MP
  - A5 overlying distal interphalangeal (DIP) joint, attached to base of distal phalanx
  - Cruciate pulleys (C1–4) lie between annular pulleys

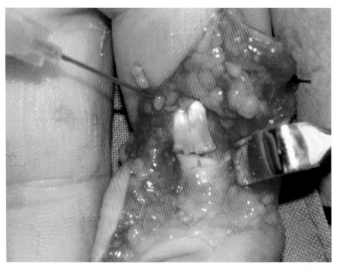

Zone 2 division of the FDP tendon to a finger. Tendon ends are approximated prior to repair. The A2 pulley can be seen just below the divided ends.

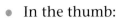

- In the thumb:
  - A1 overlying MCP joint, attached to volar plate
  - A2 overlying interphalangeal joint, attached to head of PP
  - Oblique pulley overlying shaft of PP (analogous to A2 in finger)
  - Tendon of adductor pollicis attached to A1 and oblique pulleys

What are the vinculae?

- These are vascular attachments to the flexor tendons
- Short vinculum attaches FDP to neck of MP
- Long vinculum attaches FDP to neck of PP
- FDS also has long and short vinculae both attaching to the PP

How are flexor tendon injuries managed?

- Exploration under arm tourniquet and general anaesthesia:
  - Fingers extended at the time of injury – distal ends lie in the wound
  - Fingers flexed at the time of injury – distal ends distal to the skin wound
- Operative repair preserving all pulleys and vinculae where possible:
  - Core and epitendinous sutures to allow smooth excursion of repair site through pulleys
- Careful post-operative rehabilitation in a protective splint for 6 weeks
- Tendon grafting may be necessary where presentation is delayed

Hand injuries: fractures and dislocations

Which hand fractures may be considered 'acceptable'?

- Tuft fracture of distal phalanx:
  - ◆ A tuft fracture underlying a subungal haematoma should be considered to be open
- AP displacement of metaphyseal fractures in children
- Metacarpal neck fractures:
  - ◆ <15° angulation in middle and ring fingers
  - ◆ <70° angulation in index and little fingers
- Metacarpal base fractures:
  - ◆ <20° in adults
  - ◆ <40° in children

When do hand fractures require manipulation/fixation?

- Rotational angulation
- Severe dorsal angulation
- Lateral angulation
- Shortening

What techniques are available for the stabilisation of hand fractures?

- Manipulation and stabilisation using a Plaster of Paris (PoP) splint
- Percutaneous K-wiring
- Interosseus wiring
- Lag screw fixation – spiral fractures
- Screw plus miniplate (generally only metacarpal fractures)
- External fixation – comminuted open/closed fractures

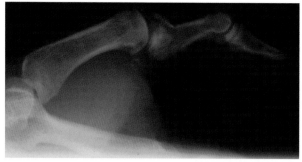

Closed fracture to the base of the proximal phalanx of the thumb.

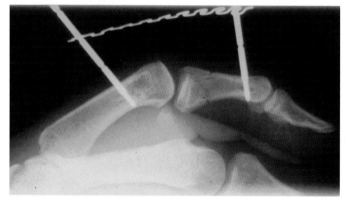

Post-reduction X-ray showing position of fragments held by S-QUATTRO external fixator.

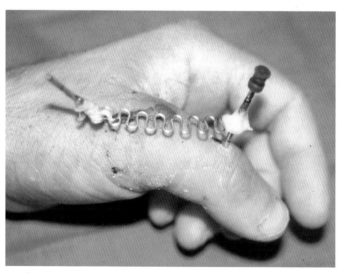

External fixator in situ.

Case Presentations in Plastic Surgery

How are joint dislocations categorised?

- Open or closed
- Simple (reduce easily) or complex (will not reduce due to soft tissue interposition)
- Fracture dislocations
- Complex dislocations more common in 'border' digits – thumb, index and little

How are hand dislocations managed?

- If closed and stable buddy strap to neighbouring digit and begin movement as pain allows
- Distal interphalangeal (DIP) joint dislocations usually easily reduced by longitudinal traction
- Proximal interphalangeal (PIP) joint dislocations commonly result in flexion contracture, permanent fusiform enlargement of the joint (mainly dorsal dislocation – volar dislocation is rare)
- Complex dislocations require open reduction and volar plate removal and repair

What is a gamekeeper's thumb?

- Hyperextension injury causing a rupture of the ulnar collateral ligament (UCL) of the metacarpophalangeal (MCP) joint, partial or total, with volar plate disruption
- Stener lesion: torn UCL lies superficial to the adductor expansion (palpable mass)
- Reattach ligament using an interosseus wire, suture or Mitec bone anchor
- Repair UCL, volar plate and dorsal capsule – all of these lend stability to the joint
- K-wire the MCP joint (6 weeks)
- A bony gamekeeper's thumb may be treated conservatively if the fracture fragment involves <15–20% of the articular surface

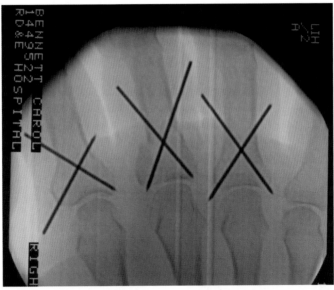

Comminuted fractures of the bases of index, middle and ring finger proximal phalanges held in reduction by crossed percutaneous K wires.

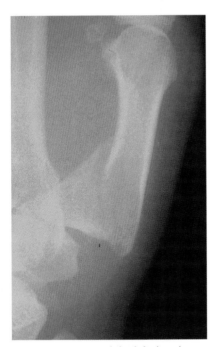

Bennett's fracture of the left thumb.

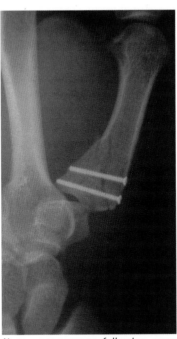

X-ray appearance following open reduction and internal screw fixation.

Case Presentations in Plastic Surgery

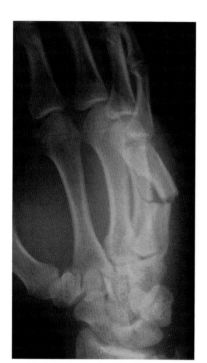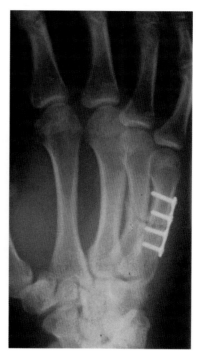

A mid shaft fracture of the fifth metacarpal treated by open reduction and internal fixation using a plate and screws.

Hand injuries: mallet deformity

What is a mallet deformity?

- Rupture of the insertion of the extensor communis tendon at the base of the distal phalanx causing extensor lag at the distal interphalangeal (DIP) joint:
  - Open due to crush/laceration injury
  - Closed due to forced flexion of the extended digit
- ? zone of relatively poor vascularity

How are mallet injuries classified?

- Type 1: Closed, with or without small avulsion fracture
- Type 2: Open
- Type 3: Open, loss of tendon substance
- Type 4:
  A: trans-epiphyseal plate fracture;
  B: fracture involving 20–50% of articular surface (hyper-flexion);
  C: hyper-extension injury >50% of articular surface, volar subluxation
- Most common type is Type 1

What is the management of a mallet deformity?

- Operative treatment of a mallet injury may downgrade flexion so treat conservatively, if possible
- Where the joint is open it should be irrigated thoroughly, non-viable tissue debrided and prophylactic antibiotics should be considered
- Type 1:
  - Stack splint 6 weeks
  - Occupational need for early return to work or poor patient compliance – consider buried K-wire

Case Presentations in Plastic Surgery

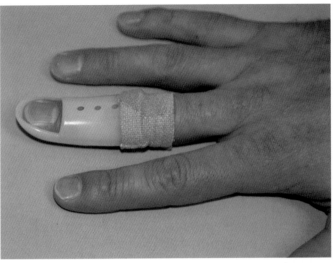

A closed mallet injury treated by simple external splintage for 6 weeks.

- Type 2:
  - ◆ Suture of tendon and skin either separately or together (tenodermodesis)
  - ◆ Stack splint 6 weeks
- Type 3:
  - ◆ Primary tendon reconstruction (distally based extensor communis flap) plus oblique K-wire to DIP joint
  - ◆ Secondary extensor reconstruction
- Type 4:
  - ◆ A: manipulation under anaesthetic plus stack splint 4 weeks
  - ◆ B and C: open reduction and K-wiring of DIP joint, maintaining reduction with pull-out suture over button on pulp; mini screw fixation
  - ◆ Some loss of active flexion in operated patients
- Other options:
  - ◆ Arthrodesis – comminuted intra-articular fracture, elderly
  - ◆ Amputation – severe soft tissue injury, devascularisation
- The proximal interphalangeal (PIP) joint is of utmost importance – keep active to avoid a Boutonniere deformity

Hand injuries: skin loss

Outline the treatment options in the management of skin loss in the hand?

- Dressings only:
  - ◆ Wound heals by secondary intention – often causing contraction of sensate skin into the defect
- Skin graft – split or full thickness:
  - ◆ Split skin graft useful in areas of relatively low vascularity and may facilitate contraction of sensate skin into the defect
- Local flap (homodigital):
  - ◆ Advancement of skin from the same digit into the defect leaving a donor site that closes directly
  - ◆ Examples include Atasoy flap, Moberg flap, Evans step advancement flap and neurosensory island flap
  - ◆ Dorsal skin defects may be reconstructed using a dorsal phalangeal island flap
- Distant flap (homodigital):
  - ◆ For example, reversed digital artery island flap
- Distant flap (heterodigital):
  - ◆ Cross finger flap:
    - ▪ Can be used to reconstruct a volar skin defect or de-epithelialised to reconstruct the dorsum
    - ▪ Disadvantaged by 'injury' to a non-traumatised digit that often becomes stiff and not suited to elderly patients
    - ▪ Pedicle divided at 2–3 weeks
  - ◆ Foucher flap – based on first dorsal metacarpal artery – can be used to reconstruct proximal defects on the dorsum of the fingers and defects on either dorsal or volar surfaces of the thumb
  - ◆ Littler flap – based upon the radial digital artery of the ring finger – used to reconstruct proximal volar defects of the fingers and thumb

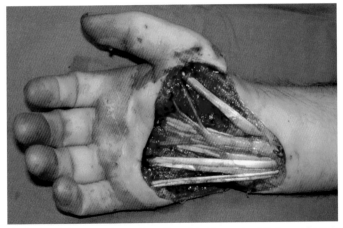

Severe degloving injury to the palm after debridement with loss of intrinsic and hypothenar musculature and exposure of tendons and branches of the median nerve.

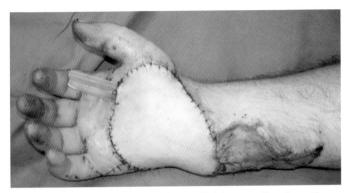

Reconstruction of palmar skin using a free radial forearm flap from the contralateral upper limb.

- Major pedicled flap:
  - Radial forearm flap, distally based, to cover large defects on the dorsal or palmar surfaces
- Free flap:
  - Contralateral radial forearm flap, lateral arm flap and anterolateral thigh flap in thin individuals
  - Toe pulp transfer to reconstruct fingertip/pulp defects
  - Toe–hand transfer (great toe used to reconstruct an amputated thumb)
- Amputation/terminalisation of a digit:
  - Shortens a digit to facilitate soft tissue cover at the tip
  - Non-replantable traumatic amputations
  - Expedites healing and return to work at the expense of length

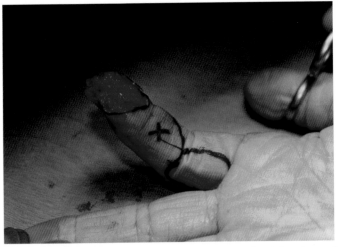

Pulp loss in the index finger. A reversed digital artery island flap is marked out from the ulnar border of the finger. 'X' marks the pivot point of the ulnar digital artery providing retrograde flow to the skin flap.

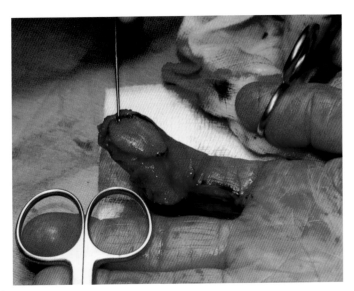

Flap inset.

Hypospadias

What is hypospadias?

- Hypospadias is characterised by ventral dystopia of the urethral meatus associated with a dorsally hooded prepuce, clefting of the glans, ventral curvature on erection (chordee) and ventral skin shortage
- May also be associated with cryptorchidism and congenital inguinal hernia
- Occurs ~1 in 300 live male births
- Hypospadias is the result of incomplete closure of the urethral folds over the urethral tube during the 12th week of embryological development
- Aetiological factors include environmental oestrogens (maternal vegetarianism), intersex states and genetic influence (familial hypospadias)

What is the pre-operative work-up for a patient with hypospadias?

- History:
  - Family history of hypospadias
  - Any urinary tract infections (UTIs) or known abnormalities of the upper genito-urinary (GU) tract
  - Any failure to thrive (UTI)
  - Maternal drugs, occupation of the father, etc.
  - Any witnessed erections – curvature?
- Examination:
  - Penis – size, degree of meatal dystopia, chordee and dorsal hooding
  - Testes – descended/undescended and size
  - Hernial orifices
- Investigations:
  - Ureas and electrolytes (U&Es), renal ultrasonographic study (USS) or isotope renogram if concerned about upper GU tract
  - Investigation of cryptorchidism or intersex states

Case Presentations in Plastic Surgery

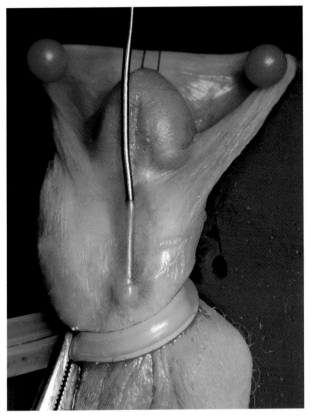

Intra-operative demonstration of proximal meatal dystopia in hypospadias. Note also dorsal hooding of the prepuce and a ventral glans groove.

What treatment is advocated for hypospadias?

- One- or two-stage surgical correction depending upon degree of deformity and operator preference
- Two-stage repair (as described by Bracka) often better able to deal with a wider spectrum of hypospadias, is technically easier, gives more reliable results, avoids a circumferential anastomosis (a potential site of stricture formation) and achieves a more natural-looking slit-like meatus
- Aims to allow micturition while standing with a non-turbulent stream, achieve a natural appearance and allow normal sexual function
- Commonly performed after 18 months of age, first and second stages separated by 6 months
- Complications include:
  - *Early*: haematoma, infection and dehiscence (all → fistulae)
  - *Late*: fistula (turbulent flow), stenosis and poor aesthetics

Keratoacanthoma

What is a keratoacanthoma?

- A rapidly evolving benign tumour which resembles a well-differentiated squamous cell carcinoma (SCC)
- If untreated within 6–8 weeks, it begins to involute
- Predominantly white races from middle age onwards
- Males > females (3×)

Clinical:

- Globular tumour
- Keratin plug or horn
- Radial symmetry
- Face and dorsum of hand

Pathology:

- Keratin-filled crypt
- Rapidly dividing squamous cells deriving from skin appendages
- Atypical mitoses and loss of polarity

What causes keratoacanthoma formation?

- Sun exposure
- Coal, tar and carcinogenic hydrocarbons (multiple lesions)
- Injury and infection including skin graft donor sites
- Association with calcium larynx, internal malignancies and leukaemia
- Association with deficient cell-mediated immunity (multiple lesions)

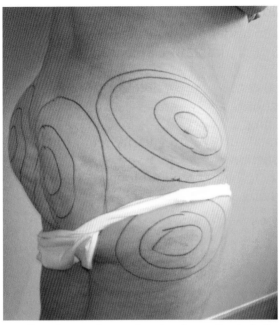

Pre-operative markings in a patient undergoing liposuction to buttocks, hips and thighs.

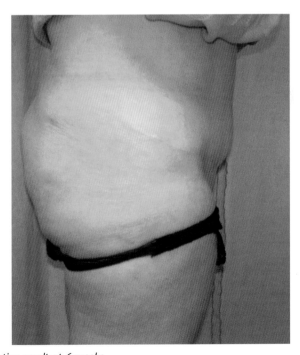

Post-operative result at 6 weeks.

Case Presentations in Plastic Surgery

What could a patient undergoing liposuction expect?

- Some pain and bruising in treated areas
- Need to wear a support garment in the post-operative period
- Potential complications of liposuction include:
    - Infection
    - Bleeding
    - Residual contour irregularity requiring further liposuction
    - Injury to nerves, major blood vessels and overlying skin

Lip reconstruction

What tumours tend to involve the lips?

- Upper lip lesions tend to be basal cell carcinomas (BCCs)
- Lower lip lesions tend to be squamous cell carcinomas (SCCs) (only 5% of SCCs occur on the upper lip)
- Commissural and mucosal SCCs have a higher propensity for metastasis
- Tumour size and thickness also correlates with metastatic potential
- May need to combine surgery with radiotherapy

How is the upper lip reconstructed?

- Loss of up to one-fourth of the upper lip may be closed directly
- Abbé flap
  - Pedicled flap from the lower lip (two-stage procedure) – lower lip shares the defect
  - Useful for central or lateral defects up to 50% of the upper lip
  - Requires an intact commissure (if commissure is absent, use Abbe–Estlander flap in one stage)
- Karapandzic flap:
  - Neurovascular flap that transfers skin, muscle and mucosa
  - Oral circumference advancement technique
  - Needs an intact commissure
  - Introduces no new tissue – hence leads to microstomia but will stretch up
  - Achieves correct muscle orientation

How can the lower lip be reconstructed?

- Ideally should remain sensate and with a good sulcus created by innervated muscle to prevent drooling

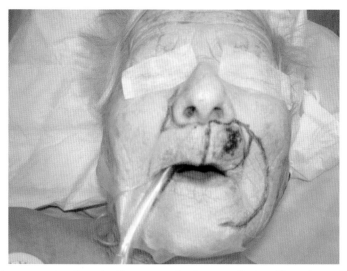

Planning reconstruction to the upper lip in a patient with a large SCC. A Karapandzic flap is marked out on the left side while an advancement flap is intended from the right side, facilitated by crescentic perialar skin excision.

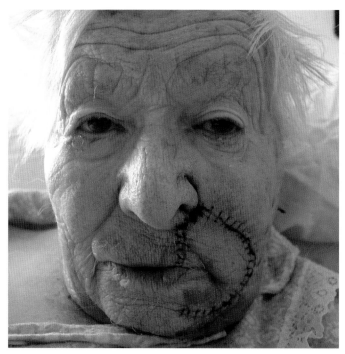

Post-operative result.

Case Presentations in Plastic Surgery

- Loss of up to one-third of the lower lip may also be closed directly
- *In situ* SCC may be treated by lip shave and mucosal advancement
- Defects one- to two-thirds of the lower lip:
  - Flaps from the upper lip as above
  - McGregor flap:
    - Myocutaneous flap
    - Rotates around the commissure
    - Commissure remains in the same place
    - Introduces new tissue into the lip to avoid microstomia
    - Lip becomes devoid of vermillion and functioning muscle but theoretical risk of drooling rarely observed
    - Vermillion may be reconstructed by mucosal advancement or tongue flap

Lower limb trauma

How are compound tibial fractures classified?

Gustillo and Anderson's compound tibial fracture classification:

I   Clean wound <1 cm
II   Wound 1–5 cm but no significant tissue disruption
IIIA Wound >5 cm but adequate soft tissue coverage with local tissues
IIIB Extensive soft tissue loss, contamination and periosteal stripping
IIIC Arterial injury requiring repair

What are the important considerations in treating patients with major limb trauma?

- Adhere to Advanced Trauma Life Support (ATLS) principles of immediate management of severe trauma
- Consider the mechanism of injury – high versus low energy
- High-energy fractures:
  - Have a poorer prognosis
  - Features in the history:
    - Road traffic accident (RTA)
    - Fall from a height
    - Missile injuries
  - Clinical signs:
    - Large/multiple wounds
    - Crush or burst lacerations
    - Closed degloving
    - Signs of nerve or vascular injury
  - Radiological signs:
    - Multiple bony fragments
    - More than one fractured bone in the same limb
    - Widely spaced fragments
    - Segmental injury

Case Presentations in Plastic Surgery

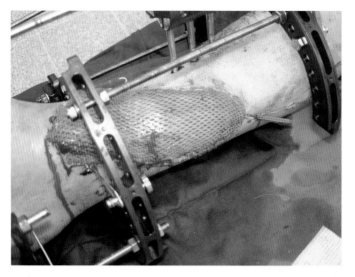

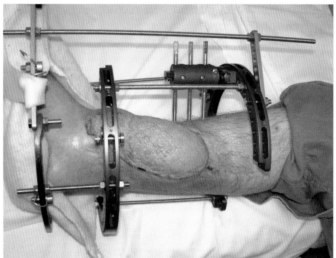

Grade IIIb fracture of the distal third of the tibia. The soft tissue defect has been reconstructed using a free rectus abdominis muscle flap. The flap, with a meshed skin graft, is shown at the end of the reconstruction (top) and at 6 weeks (bottom).

- Determining salvagability of the limb:
  - ◆ Is revascularisation needed?
  - ◆ Is the soft tissue defect reconstructable?
  - ◆ Is there any bone loss?
    - ■ Is this reconstructable?
  - ◆ Is there any nerve injury?
    - ■ Results of nerve repair and grafting in the lower limb are poor except in children
- Reconstructive plan:
  1 Debridement of all non-viable tissue and pulsed lavage under tourniquet
  2 Reduce and stabilise the fracture
  3 Restore perfusion by arterial reconstruction, if necessary
  4 Fasciotomy
  5 Stable, well-vascularised soft tissue cover, e.g. free muscle flap

Lymphoedema

What is lymphoedema?

- The accumulation of protein-rich interstitial fluid in subcutaneous (s.c.) tissues
  - Women > men; left leg > right leg and lower limb > upper limb

How is lymphoedema classified?

- Primary:
  - At birth (Milroy's disease) or <14 years
  - Adolescence (lymphoedema praecox) or 14–35 years, 80% of all cases
  - Later in life (lymphoedema tarda) or >35 years
- Secondary:
  - Neoplastic – malignant nodes, extrinsic compression of lymphatics
  - Infective – tuberculosis (TB), *Wucheria bancrofti*
  - Iatrogenic – lymphadenectomy and radiotherapy

What is the pathogenesis of lymphoedema?

- Leakage of protein into the interstitium → raised tissue oncotic pressure → increased interstitial protein and fluid → tissue hypoxia → cell death → chronic inflammatory response → fibrosis

How does lymphoedema present?

- Initially pitting then non-pitting oedema and skin ulceration due to fibrosis
- Lymphangiosarcoma may develop >10 years (poor prognosis)

What investigations are conducted for lymphoedema?

- Exclude deep vein thrombosis (DVT) (doppler/venogram)
- Image the pelvic nodes for tumours

Case Presentations in Plastic Surgery

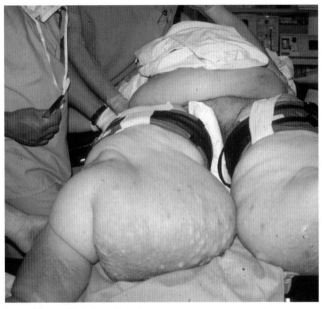

Severe bilateral lower limb lymphoedema.

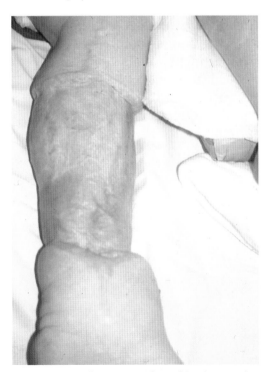

Appearance following excisional surgery with grafting in a patient with moderate lymphoedema.

Case Presentations in Plastic Surgery

- Exclude hepatic, renal or cardiac causes
- Lymphangiography

How is lymphoedema treated?

- Remove the precipitating cause if secondary:
  1 Medical:
     - Skin care – prevention of ulceration
     - Treatment of lymphangitis and cellulitis
     - Elevation, foot pumps, complex regional physiotherapy and compression garments
  2 Excisional surgery (indicated in <10%):
     - Excision of all soft tissue down to fascia and skin graft (Charles)
     - Excision of s.c. lymphoedematous tissue preserving overlying skin flaps (Homan)
     - Excision of s.c. tissue and burying of a dermal flap into the uninvolved muscle compartment (Thompson):
       - Creates a theoretical lymphatic communication allowing drainage of the skin via the deep compartment
  3 Physiological surgery:
     - Rarely successful
     - Microsurgical lympho-venous and lympho-lymphatic shunts

Malignant melanoma

What is a malignant melanoma?

- A malignant tumour of epidermal melanocytes
- Affects young adults, female:male ratio 2:1, in Celtic and Caledonian races
- Incidence around 6 per 100 000 per year in the UK, increasing especially in men
- <5% of all skin cancers, but >75% of skin cancer deaths

What factors have been implicated in the aetiology of malignant melanoma?

- Short intense episodes of sun exposure (ultra violet rays B, UVB) and sunburn in childhood
- Premalignant lesions including dysplastic naevi and non-invasive lentigo maligna
- Genetic predisposition, e.g. xeroderma pigmentosa
- <10% arise in pre-existing naevi, lifetime risk of giant congenital naevus <4%

How do melanomas present?

- History of growth in a pre-existing mole, darkening, itching, ulceration and bleeding
- Variegated pigmentation; typically a haphazard array of brown-black pigmentation
- Asymmetry: irregular border and surface

What types of melanoma are there?

- Superficial spreading:
  - ◆ 50–70% of all melanomas
  - ◆ Flat, irregular border, pigmentation and surface
- Nodular:
  - ◆ 10–20% of all melanomas, concurrent radial and vertical growth

Case Presentations in Plastic Surgery

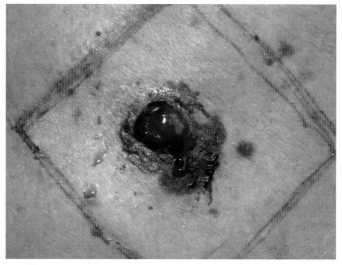

Nodular malignant melanoma.

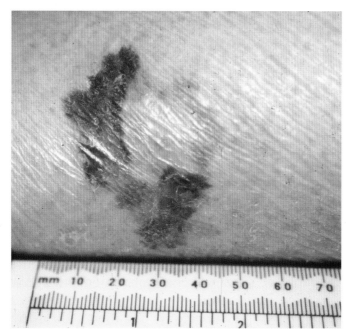

Superficial spreading malignant melanoma.

- Lentigo maligna melanoma (Hutchinson's melanotic freckle):
  - Sun-exposed skin, especially face, of older patients, women > men
  - 5–10% of all melanomas; invasive change in a lentigo maligna (30–50%)
- Acral lentiginous melanoma:
  - Palms, soles and mucocutaneous junctions
  - 2–8% of melanomas in Caucasians but up to 60% in dark-skinned races
  - Subungal: great toe affected in around 50% of cases, thumb the next most common
- Secondary melanoma (no identifiable primary):
  - Accounts for around 5% of melanomas
  - Usually present as lymph node disease, also skin, brain and lung
- Desmoplastic melanoma (desmoplastic-spindling stroma):
  - Most commonly in the head and neck, high local but low nodal recurrence

What prognostic indicators are there for melanoma?

- Depth (Breslow) and level (Clark) of invasion into the skin
- Ulceration, high mitotic rate and positive sentinel node biopsy lead to poorer prognosis

How are melanomas managed?

- Excision biopsy followed by wide local excision with or without sentinel node biopsy
- Additional staging investigations including computerised tomography (CT) scan of chest, abdomen and pelvis
- Observation for local or regional (nodal) recurrence or completion lymphadenectomy in patients following positive sentinel node biopsy
- Adjuvant chemotherapy within the context of clinical trials

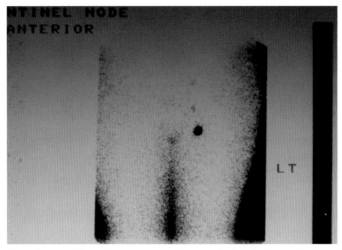

Sentinel lymph node biopsy in melanoma. The sentinel node is the first lymph gland to which dermal lymphatics carry an isotope of Technitium, injected intradermally at the site of excision biopsy of the primary tumour and imaged pre-operatively using a gamma camera. This lymphoscintgram has identified a groin sentinel node in a patient with a lower limb primary malignant melanoma.

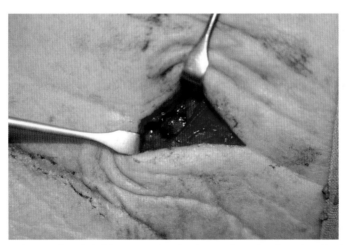

At operation, a hand held gamma probe is used to localise the 'hot' node. Identification is assisted by visualisation of the gland using dye, similarly injected at the biopsy site. In this patient, a level III cervical sentinel node has been identified using this 'double hit' technique. The sentinel node is removed and examined carefully for the presence of occult microscopic nodal disease. If positive, early regional nodal clearance can be undertaken.

Case Presentations in Plastic Surgery

Mandible reconstruction

How is the mandible affected by intra-oral tumours?

- Most intra-oral tumours involve bone
- Access to excision of intra-oral tumours may require splitting the mandible
- >90% of intra-oral tumours are squamous cell carcinoma (SCC)
- Invasion of the dentate mandible is heralded by loosening of teeth
- Bone changes secondary to radiotherapy are difficult to distinguish from tumour
- Trismus (pterygoid involvement) and pain radiating to the ear or temple (auriculotemporal nerve) or lower lip (mental nerve) are poor prognostic signs

What are the principles of mandible resection?

- Choice between rim resection and segmental resection
- Rim resection only feasible in the non-irradiated mandible for early tumour
- T3 or T4 tumours may require segmental resection
- Virtually all mandibular resections are accompanied by synchronous neck dissection whether or not there is palpable disease

What are the aims of mandible reconstruction?

- Enable normal chewing and swallowing
- Maintain oral competence
- Denture rehabilitation
- Aesthetics

How is mandible reconstruction achieved?

- Non-vascularised bone grafts:
  - Bone segment iliac crest or rib grafts
  - Particulate bone and cancellous marrow (PBCM)
  - Complicated by resorption

Case Presentations in Plastic Surgery

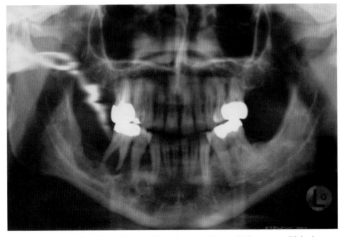

Orthopantomogram showing right sided destruction of the mandible by tumour.

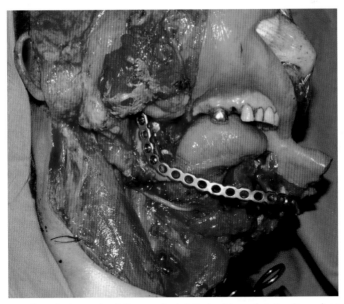

Intra-operative photograph of the surgical defect with a plate in situ *prior to insetting of a deep circumflex iliac artery (DCIA) osseocutaneous flap.*

Case Presentations in Plastic Surgery

- Pedicled osteomyocutaneous flaps
  - Trapezius/spine of scapula
  - Pectoralis major/fifth rib or edge of sternum
- Free vascularised bone flaps:
  - Radial forearm flap
  - Iliac crest free flap
  - Free fibula flap
  - Scapula flap
  - Flaps can incorporate a skin paddle for external and/or mucosal reconstruction
  - Consider osseointegration of teeth – depends upon bone volume
- Alloplastic materials:
  - Bone substitutes (such as hydroxyapatite) are rigid, cannot support a prosthesis and do not remodel
  - Metal plates may be used as a temporary support only

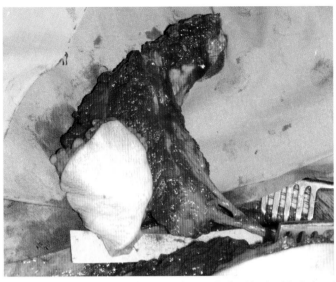

DCIA flap raised on its pedicle. (Photograph supplied with the kind permission of Mr J Palmer.)

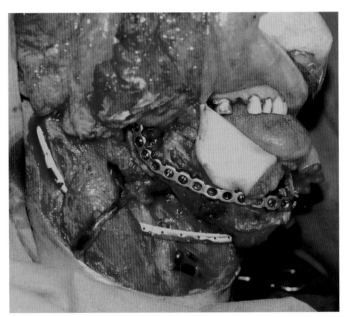

Flap inset. The venous anastomosis can be seen overlying the sternocleidomastoid muscle. (Photograph supplied with the kind permission of Mr J Palmer.)

Case Presentations in Plastic Surgery

Nasal reconstruction

What are the aims of nasal reconstruction?
- Provide good cosmesis
- Ensure a patent airway
- Reconstruction of skin, support and lining

How is skin reconstruction achieved?
- Full thickness skin grafts
- Composite grafts:
  - Skin and cartilage
  - Skin and fat
- Local flaps:
  - Median glabellar advancement flap
  - Bilobed flap
  - Nasolabial flap either one- or two-stage procedure
  - V–Y flaps from the cheek
  - Forehead flap:
    - Based on supratrochlear vessels
    - May be taken high into the scalp in male pattern baldness
    - Subperiosteal dissection from a point 2 cm above the supraorbital rim to the medial canthus to preserve supratrochlear vessels
  - Scalping rhinoplasty (converse):
    - Based laterally on superficial temporal vessels
    - Makes use of 60–70% of the whole forehead, arching into anterior scalp
  - Pedicle divided after 2–3 weeks
- Free flaps:
  - Radial forearm flap
  - May include bone

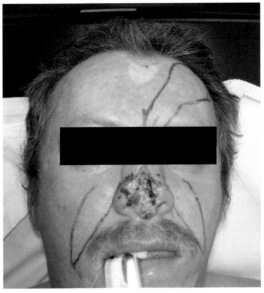

Patient with extensive recurrent BCC of the nose prior to excisional surgery with histological control of margins.

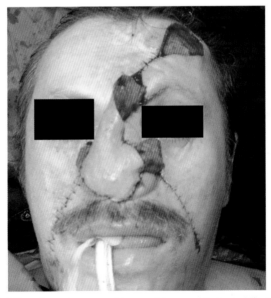

Two nasolabial flaps have been used to provide nasal lining while a forehead flap has been used for nasal skin reconstruction. Pedicles are divided at approximately 3 weeks. Further surgery to refine nasal cosmesis can be undertaken at later stages.

Case Presentations in Plastic Surgery

How is the lining of the nose reconstructed?

- In-turning of pedicled forehead flaps
- Skin grafts to the inner raw surface of pedicled forehead flaps
- In-turning of external nasal skin
- Nasolabial flaps

How is the support to the nose achieved?

- Ideally provided at the same time as skin/lining reconstruction
- Mid-line support:
  - ◆ L-shaped costochondral strut from the nasal radix and angulated to contact the anterior nasal spine but produces a wide columella
  - ◆ Cantilever bone graft screwed to the nasal radix to provide projection

What other reconstructive options are available?

- Branemark osseintegrated prosthesis
- Prosthesis suspended on spectacles

Necrotising fasciitis

What organisms are implicated in necrotising fasciitis?
- Mixed anaerobe and Group A streptococcal infection:
  - Group A *Streptococcus* carried in nose/throat of 15% of the population
- Pathogenesis – production of:
  - Pyrogenic toxins
  - Haemolysins
  - Hyaluronidase
  - Streptokinase

What are the risk factors for necrotising fasciitis?
- Insulin-dependent diabetes mellitus (IDDM)
- Minor trauma/surgery
- Non-steroidal anti-inflammatory drugs (NSAIDs) (most correlation)
- *Varicella zoster* virus infections

How does necrotising fasciitis present?
- Local swelling, redness and intense pain
- Dusky hue, areas of purple necrosis and blistering
- Very rapid extension of skin changes
- Systemic toxicity:
  - Apathy
  - Confusion
  - Septic shock
  - Elderly may be unable to mount a pyrexia
- Mortality up to 53%

How is necrotising fasciitis managed?
- High-dose intravenous (i.v.) antibiotics
  - For example, clindamycin (also stops the production of toxins) and imipenem

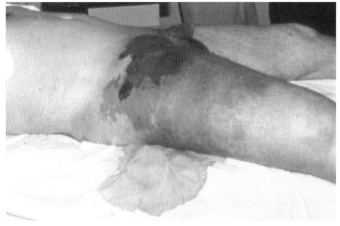

Skin changes typical of necrotising fasciits.

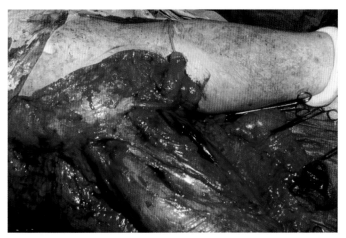

Debridement of necrotic skin, subcutaneous fat and fascia revealed necrotising myositis in this patient. A hind quarter amputation was therefore undertaken.

- Emergency radical surgical debridement
- Intensive therapy unit (ITU) supportive therapy
  - Ventilation/oxygenation
  - Inotropic support where necessary
  - Dialysis

How does necrotising fasciitis compare with gas gangrene?

- Similar onset, sick patient
- Surgical emphysema (crepitus)
- Bloody blisters: aspirate → *Clostridium welchii* (Gram-negative bacillus)
- Aggressive surgical approach
- Some evidence to support the role of hyperbaric oxygen
- High mortality

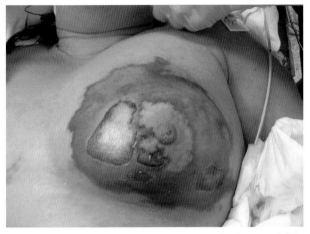

Necrotising fasciitis of the breast prior to immediate radical surgical debridement.

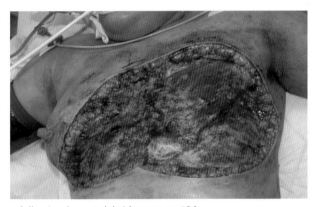

Appearance following breast debridement at 48 h.

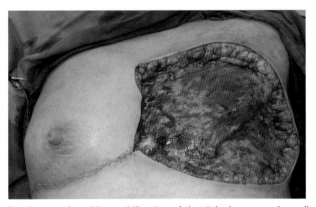

The defect has been reduced by mobilisation of the right breast and a split skin graft can be used to close the wound prior to staged breast reconstruction.

Case Presentations in Plastic Surgery

Neurofibromatosis

What is neurofibromatosis-1 (NF-1)?

- Autosomal-dominant inheritance, incidence 1 in 3000
- Multiple cutaneous neurofibromas (proliferating Schwann cells and fibroblasts)
- *Café au lait* patches (>5 is abnormal)
- Axillary freckles
- Iris hamartomas (Lisch nodules)

What may be associated with NF-1?

- Neural:
  - Optic nerve glioma
  - Meningioma
  - Plexiform neurofibroma
  - Phaeochromocytoma
  - Neurofibromas may undergo sarcomatous change
  - Mental retardation
- Cardiovascular:
  - Orbital haemangioma
  - Renal artery stenosis
  - Obstructive cardiomyopathy
  - Also pulmonary fibrosis
- Bony:
  - Scoliosis, fibrous dysplasia

What is neurofibromatosis-2 (NF-2)?

- NF-2 is less common, separate gene defect (Alzheimer's disease, AD) and is associated with acoustic neuroma

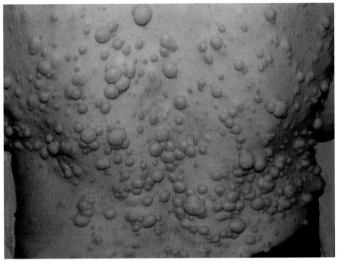

Multiple cutaneous neurofibromas in a patient with type 1 neurofibromatosis.

Oral tumours

What type of tumours occur within the mouth?

- >90% of intra-oral tumours are squamous cell carcinoma (SCC)
- Sublingual and minor mucosal salivary glands form high-grade adenoid cystic tumours
- Acral lentiginous melanoma of oral mucosa
- Sarcomas
- *Synchronous* tumours – detected within 6 months – up to 15%
- *Metachronous* tumours – detected beyond 6 months

How are intra-oral tumours managed?

- Examination under anaesthesia (EUA) is often necessary to establish the degree of spread within the mouth
- Magnetic resonance imaging (MRI), including the neck and nodes, also helpful
- T1 and low-volume T2 tumours of the floor of the mouth can be reasonably treated by brachytherapy alone, if their distance from the mandible will avoid radionecrosis
- Total glossectomy mainly reserved for:
  - T3/T4 tumours
  - Post-radiotherapy recurrence
  - Cases where >50% of the tongue is involved
- T1 tongue tumours demand excision, but no neck dissection
- T2 tongue tumours usually demand ipsilateral neck dissection
- T2 tumours of the *tip* of the tongue usually demand bilateral neck dissection (35% incidence of occult nodal disease in the N0 neck)
- T4 tumours show involvement of extrinsic muscles of the tongue

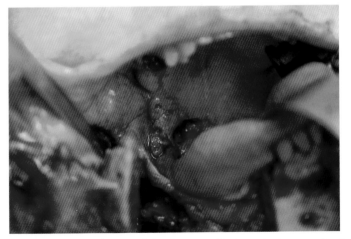

A tonsillar fossa SCC can be seen following mandibular osteotomy and extraction of upper and lower molar teeth.

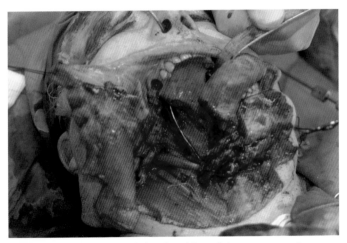

The surgical defect created by wide local excision of the tumour and supraomohyoid neck dissection.

What reconstructive options are available following total glossectomy?

- Pectoralis major myocutaneous flap
- Myocutaneous free flap – need bulk

How are defects of the floor of mouth reconstructed?

- Allow small defects to granulate
- Primary closure
- Flap closure:
  - Tunnelled nasolabial flaps
  - Pectoralis major myocutaneous flap
  - Temporalis muscle flap
  - Temporoparietal fascial flap
  - Free flap, e.g. radial forearm flap

What other factors are important when managing patients with head and neck cancers?

- Airway management (tracheostomy)
- Avoid neck tapes
- Post-operative speech therapy
- Post-operative nasogastric tube (NGT) feeding
- Infection prophylaxis
- Psychological support
- Pain management

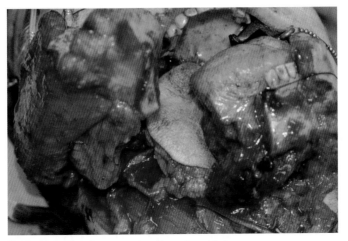

Free radial forearm flap for reconstruction of oral lining.

Osteoarthritis of the basal joint of the thumb

Which is the most commonly affected joint of osteoarthritis (OA)?

- The most common joint to be affected by OA is the first carpo-metacarpal joint

How is the pain associated with basal joint OA graded?

- Arnot and Saint Laurent:
  - 0 No pain
  - 1 Pain during particular activities
  - 2 Pain during daily activities
  - 3 Episodes of spontaneous pain
  - 4 Constant pain

What other features OA may be visible in a patient with basal joint disease?

- Heberden's nodes: osteophytes at the distal interphalangeal (DIP) joint
- Bouchard's nodes: osteophytes at the proximal interphalangeal (PIP) joint

How are the radiological signs staged?

- I Less than one-third subluxation at carpo-metacarpal joint
- II Greater than one-third subluxation, osteophytes
- III Sclerosis, joint space narrowing and osteophytes >2 mm
- IV Advanced degenerative changes, also involving scaphotrapezial joint

What are the treatment options?

- Carpo-metacarpal joint splinting
- Intra-articular steroids

Case Presentations in Plastic Surgery

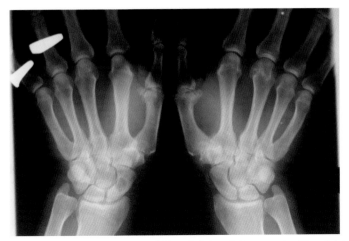

Osteoarthritis of the carpometacarpal (basal) joint of the thumbs. The right side is severely affected (radiological grade 4) showing loss of joint space, subluxation, osteophyte formation and degenerative changes in the scaphotrapezial joint.

- Basal osteotomy (a wedge osteotomy, removing the radial cortex of the metacarpal to change the vector of stress forces acting on the joint)
- Trapeziectomy
- Joint replacement
- Arthrodesis

Pressure sores

What is a pressure sore?

- The breakdown of skin and underlying soft tissue due to unrelieved pressure-induced ischaemia in non-ambulatory patients or in patients with a sensory neuropathy
- Pure pressure sores begin with tissue necrosis deep near the bony prominence leading to a cone-shaped area of tissue breakdown with its apex at the skin surface
- Worsening this situation is the soft tissue damage caused by moisture, infection and shear forces

How are pressure sores graded?

1 Erythema
2 Blistering
3 Subcutaneous (s.c.) muscle breakdown
4 Bone/joint involvement

What are the common sites for pressure sore formation?

- Supine patient: sacral and heel sores
- Sitting: ischial sores
- Lying on one side: trochanteric sores

How are patients with pressure sores managed?

- General:
  - Optimise nutrition
  - Correct anaemia
  - Prevention and treatment of infection
  - Catheterise to avoid exposure to moisture
  - Treatment of contractures – BoTox, tenotomy and amputation
  - Use of pressure-relieving beds/matresses
  - Relieve pressure by regular turning

Case Presentations in Plastic Surgery

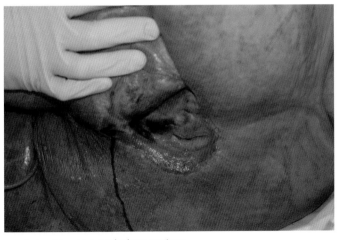

Large sacral sore in a non-ambulant patient.

- Dressings to encourage healing from the base
- Surgery:
  - Debridement of the sore
  - Excision of bony prominences, often necrotic
  - Wound closure with healthy tissues, often in the form of local rotation or transposition flaps

Ptosis

What is eyelid ptosis?

- Normal lid level is covering 1–2 mm of the upper limbus of the iris
- Ptosis is an abnormal droopiness of the upper lid

How is ptosis classified?

- *Congenital*:
  - ◆ Absence of levator
  - ◆ Lid lag commonly accompanies a congenital ptosis
  - ◆ Leave alone until ~5 years unless:
    1 Severe ptosis obstructing visual field leading to amblyopia
    2 Corneal exposure risking ulceration
- *Acquired*:
  - ◆ Neurogenic:
    - Occulomotor necrosis lesion (levator palpebrae superioris)
    - Horner's syndrome (correct with 10% phenylephrine hydrochloride)
    - Demyelination
    - Traumatic ophthalmoplegia or ophthalmoplegic migraine
  - ◆ *Myogenic*:
    - Senile ptosis – stretching of the levator aponeurosis and muscle with age
    - Myaesthenia gravis (tensilon test)
    - Muscular dystrophy
    - Steroid ptosis
  - ◆ *Traumatic*:
    - Injury to levator mechanism
    - Also post-cataract surgery – damage to superior rectus muscle – used for insertion of a stay stitch to immobilise the eye leads to scarring

Case Presentations in Plastic Surgery

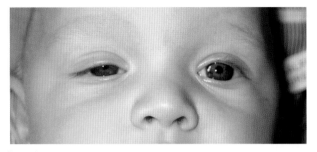

Congenital ptosis.

- ◆ *Mechanical*:
  - ■ Lid tumour
  - ■ Dermatochalasis (excess redundant skin)
- ◆ *Pseudoptosis*:
  - ■ The appearance of ptosis rather than true ptosis, e.g. with enophthalmos

How is ptosis treated?
- Depends upon the severity of the ptosis
- Plication of levator aponeurosis or shortening/plication of muscle itself
- Use of fascial slings to connect frontalis to the tarsal plate

Rheumatoid arthritis of the hand

What are the stages and pattern of rheumatoid disease?

- Stages:
  1. *Proliferative*: synovial swelling, pain, restricted movement and nerve compression
  2. *Destructive*: tendon rupture, capsular disruption, joint subluxation and bone erosion
  3. *Reparative*: fibrosis, tendon adhesions, fibrous ankylosis and fixed deformity
- Pattern:
  - *Monocyclic*: one episode, spontaneous remission, 10%
  - *Polycyclic*: remissions and relapses, 45%
  - *Progressive*: inexorable course, 45%

How are the soft tissues of the hand affected by rheumatoid arthritis?

- Synovitis:
  - Autoimmune: rheumatoid factor is a circulating macroglobulin in 70% of patients
  - Synovial inflammation, formation of pannus and erosive enzymes
  - Tender boggy swelling dorsum of wrist and around flexor tendons in the carpal canal leading to tendon ruptures and disruption of the stabilising structures around joints
- Rheumatoid nodules:
  - Fibrinoid necrosis mainly on the ulnar border of forearm (a poor prognostic sign)
- Tendon ruptures:
  - May be due to synovitis, e.g. extensor communis and horn sign

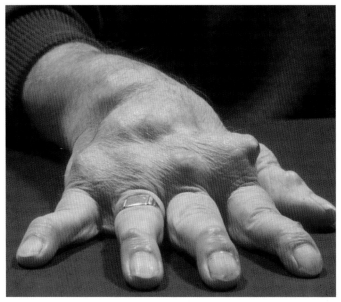

The soft tissue deformities in rheumatoid arthritis: dorsal synovitis, rheumatoid nodules, and swan necking.

- ◆ Attrition ruptures, e.g. ulnar head (extensor digiti minimi, EDM; extensor digitorum communis, EDC), scaphoid tubercle (flexor pollicis longus, FPL) and Lister's tubercle (extensor pollicis longus, EPL)
- Nerve compression:
  - ◆ Carpal tunnel syndrome

How are the joints of the hand affected by rheumatoid arthritis?

- Ulnar head syndrome:
  - ◆ Prominent ulnar head due to disruption of radioulnar (RU) ligament and distal RU joint (DRUJ) instability
  - ◆ Supination of the carpus with volar subluxation of extensor carpi ulnaris (ECU) allowing radial wrist deviation
- Wrist joint:
  - ◆ Supinated, radially deviated and volarly subluxed due to ligamentous and capsular erosion, joints grossly deranged
- Metacarpophalangeals (MCPs):
  - ◆ Ulnar drift and volar subluxation of the base of proximal phalanx
- Fingers:
  - ◆ Telescoping
  - ◆ Swan neck and Boutonniere deformity

What type of surgical intervention may be required?

- Only indicated where there is pain and loss of function
- Preventative procedures, e.g. synovectomy
- Reconstructive procedures, e.g. tendon transfers
- Salvage procedures, e.g. joint surgery including lower-end ulna excision, replacement of MCP joints (Swanson) and joint fusions; address proximal joints before distal ones

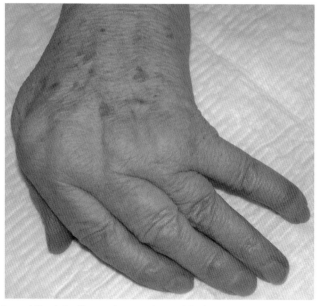

Typical ulnar drift of the fingers in a patient with rheumatoid arthritis.

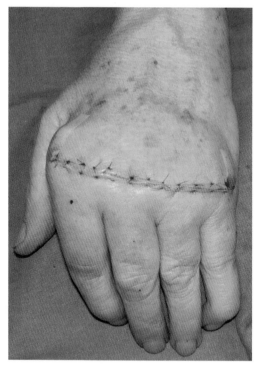

Correction of ulnar drift following MCP joint replacements using Swanson prostheses.

Case Presentations in Plastic Surgery

Rhinoplasty

What details should be elicited from the history?
- Age and occupation
- What is wrong?
- What would you like to do and why do you want to have it done?
- Any previous trauma or surgery to the nose
- Any history of nosebleeds or allergic rhinitis
- Headaches
- Olfactory disturbances
- Drugs, e.g. aspirin, warfarin and steroids
- PMSH, e.g. diabetes, hypertension, etc.
- Smoker?

What aspects of the examination are important in patients requesting a rhinoplasty?
- General shape and symmetry of the face
- Scars/swellings on the face and nose
- Mandibular hypoplasia and malocclusion
- Dorsum: deviation, width and hump
- Upper lateral cartilages: deviation, hump and supra-tip deformity
- Lower lateral (alar) cartilages/tip: width, size, hanging, pinched and valving
- Columella: size, deviation and angle (men 90°, women 100°)
- Internally: airway occlusion/septal deviation, valving (internal valve), prominence of the nasal spine

What can a patient undergoing rhinoplasty expect?
- Surgery conducted under general anaesthesia
- Painful nose
- Black eyes
- Plaster of Paris (PoP) for 1 week

Case Presentations in Plastic Surgery

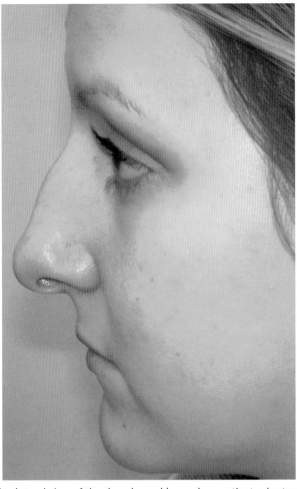

Pre-operative lateral view of the dorsal nasal hump in a patient prior to rhinoplasty.

- Nasal packs removed at 24 h
- Swollen initially but will settle
- Potential complications:
  - Intra-operative:
    - Cribiform plate fracture
    - Excessive bleeding
  - Early post-operative:
    - Infection
    - Haematoma
    - Nosebleeds (do not blow)
  - Late post-operative:
    - Residual deformity – under-correction
    - New deformity – over-correction
    - Resorption of grafts
- Scar at base of columella (open approach)

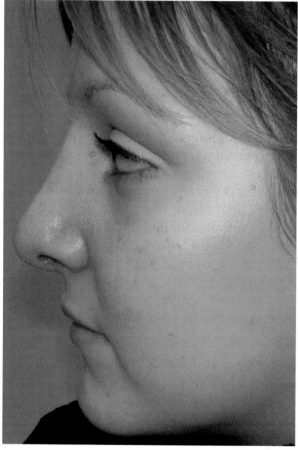

Correction of the dorsal hump following dorsal nasal osteotomy, reduction of the septum and upper lateral cartilages, and lateral maxillary osteotomy with in-fracture.

Salivary gland tumours

What are the general features of salivary gland tumours?

- Present as a localised painless nodule:
  - Pain and facial nerve involvement (weakness) strong indicators of malignancy
- 80% of all tumours are of the parotid (75% are pleomorphic adenomas)
- 10% arise in submandibular gland (65% pleomorphic adenomas and 16% adenoid cystic)
- The smaller the gland the more likely that a tumour is malignant and aggressive
- Fine needle biopsy generally safe, open biopsy risks seeding a pleomorphic adenoma

How are salivary gland tumours classified?

- Monomorphic adenoma (adenolymphoma and Warthin tumour):
  - Mainly in males >50 years
  - May be multifocal or bilateral (15%)
- Pleomorphic adenoma:
  - Slow growth
  - Incomplete excision or seeding leads to recurrence
- Myoepithelioma:
  - Occurs in minor glands causing a large intra-oral swelling
- Mucoepidermoid tumour:
  - Low- to high-grade malignancy (tends to be low grade in the major glands)
  - In the minor glands behave more like adenoid cystic carcinoma
- Carcinoma (epithelial tumours):
  - Adenoid cystic carcinoma:
    - Slow rate of growth and high local recurrence
  - Adenocarcinoma

Case Presentations in Plastic Surgery

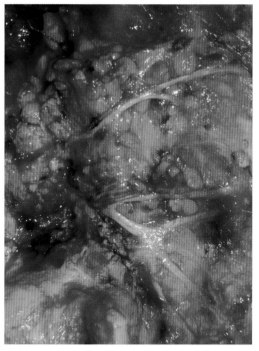

A superficial parotidectomy has been performed, carefully preserving branches of the facial nerve.

- ◆ Squamous carcinoma (often metastatic)
- ◆ Anaplastic carcinoma
- ◆ Carcinoma in pleomorphic adenoma:
  - ▪ Sudden increase in rate of growth of a long-standing lump
  - ▪ Development of fixity, facial nerve weakness or paralysis
  - ▪ Behaves like anaplastic carcinoma with a poor prognosis
- ● Malignant lymphomas

How are parotid tumours treated?

- ● Benign or low-grade parotid tumours treated by superficial parotidectomy
- ● High-grade tumour by radical parotidectomy, facial nerve graft and radiotherapy
- ● Management of neck nodes

What is Frey's syndrome?

- ● Gustatory sweating in 10–40% of patients having undergone parotidectomy
- ● Traumatised parasympathetic branches to the parotid gland degenerate to the level the cell bodies in the otic ganglion and regenerate along the auriculotemporal nerve
- ● These link up with sweat glands in the temple where eating induces sweating
- ● Treatment with antiperspirants, dermo-fat grafts and tympanic neurectomy

Scars: hypertrophic and keloid

What types of abnormal scars are there?

- Hypertrophic scars:
  - Limited to the initial boundary of the injury
  - Occur soon after injury
  - Spontaneous regression over years
  - Related to wound tension and delayed healing
  - Pull in multiple directions – hypertrophic scar
  - Pull in one direction – stretched scar
  - Sites of predilection include anterior chest, shoulders and deltoid
- Keloid scars:
  - Extension beyond the original boundary
  - Occur later after injury (months)
  - No regression
  - Better correlated with dark skin colour ($15\times$ more common in blacks)
  - Young age
  - Significant familial tendency
  - Wounds do not have to be under tension – face and earlobes may also be affected in addition to the above

What are the cellular mechanisms promoting hypertrophic and keloid scars?

- Abnormality of collagen metabolism, i.e. increased synthesis or decreased degradation
- Fibroplasia into the 3rd week without resolution
- ? sustained levels of tumour growth factor beta (TGF-b) (ratio of TGF-b1 and -2 to TGF-b3)
- High content of type III collagen, numerous Langerhans cells and vascular sensitivity symptoms due to the release of neuropeptides from nerve endings in the scar (substance P, neuropeptide Y and calcitonin gene-related peptide, CGRP)

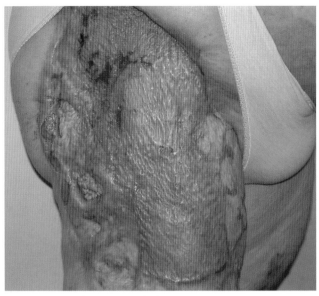

Post-burn scar hypertrophy on the right hip.

How are hypertrophic and keloid scars managed?

- Moisturising massage
- Axasain cream contains capsaicin which neutralises substance P to reduce symptoms of itching/burning
- Intralesional steroid
- Topical silicone
- Intralesional excisional surgery (may be contemplated in conjunction with post-operative radiotherapy)
- Operating on hypertrophic or keloid scars carries a significant risk of recurrence with a worse scar

Skin flaps

How are skin flaps classified?

- A random pattern flap is a flap which relies for its vascularity upon the vessels of the dermal and subdermal plexuses of the skin
- An axial pattern flap is one which is vascularised by vessels running longitudinally within it:
  - Direct cutaneous artery
  - Fasciocutaneous artery
  - Septocutaneous artery
  - Intermuscular septal perforators
  - Muscle perforators

How do skin flaps move to reconstruct a defect?

- Flaps which move about a pivot point:
  - Rotation flap:
    - A semi-circular flap which rotates about a pivot point through an arc of rotation into an adjacent defect
    - Donor site either closes directly or with a skin graft
  - Transposition flap:
    - A triangular, square or rectangular flap which moves laterally about a pivot point into an adjacent defect
  - Interpolation:
    - A flap which moves laterally about a pivot point into a defect which is not immediately adjacent to it
- Advancement flaps
  - A flap which moves forwards without rotation or lateral movement

What is a Z-plasty?

- A technique involving the transposition of two adjacent triangular flaps:
  - All limbs of the Z must be of equal length

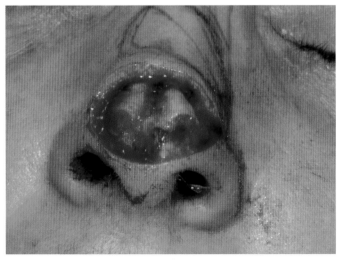

The defect created by wide local excision of a BCC on the nasal tip. The lower lateral cartilages are clearly seen in the base of the defect.

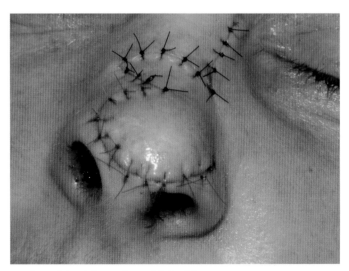

Reconstruction of the defect using a bilobed flap.

Case Presentations in Plastic Surgery

- Angles do not have to be the same
- At the completion of the transposition, the Z has been rotated by 90°

When is a Z-plasty required?

1 To transpose normal tissue into a critical area:
   - Return a vermillion step into alignment
2 To change the direction of a scar:
   - Break up an ugly scar contour on the face
   - Re-orientate a scar around the knee
3 To lengthen a scar:
   - Burn scar contracture, lip lengthening with the Tennison cleft repair

Skin grafts

What are the different types of skin grafts?

- Split skin graft:
  - Tangential excision of skin to superficial or mid-dermal level using a dermatome (air or battery driven) or Watson knife
  - Good graft take
  - Can be meshed to increase surface area, allow better conformity and prevent haematoma
  - More contraction at the recipient bed
  - Less donor site morbidity
- Full thickness skin graft:
  - Skin graft raised at dermo-fat junction
  - Retains colour and hair-bearing qualities
  - Less contracture
  - Less guaranteed take
  - Closure of donor site with a linear scar

How do skin grafts 'take'?

- Adherence:
  - Fibrin bond between graft and bed (especially if the bed is composed of granulation tissue)
- Plasmic imbibition:
  - Absorption of interstitial fluid by osmosis contributes to graft nutrition
- Revascularisation:
  - Circulation restored after 4–7 days (thicker grafts take longer)
  - Vascular connections differentiate into afferent and efferent vessels
- Maturation:
  - Increased mitoses from day 3 onwards
  - Epidermal hyperplasia (scaling and desquamation)
  - Regeneration of appendages – sweat glands and hair follicles

Case Presentations in Plastic Surgery

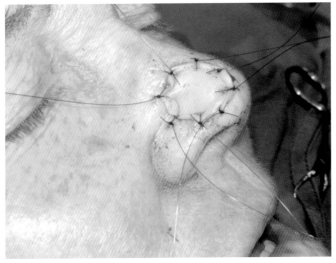

Full thickness skin graft reconstruction of a nasal defect.

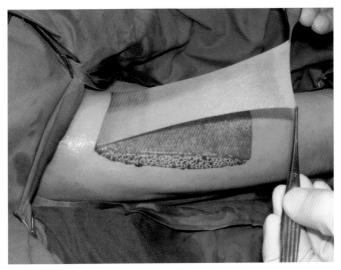

Split thickness skin graft harvested from the anterior thigh using an air-powered dermatome.

How are skin grafts inset?

- Jelonet or mepitel applied over the graft
- Tie-over dressing or sponge foam to provide splintage or compression
- Sutures or staples
- Glue
  - 2-Octyl Cyanoacrylate (**DERMABOND**)
    - applied at the margins of the graft
    - facilitates epithelical closure with or without dermal sutures at other wound sites
    - provides a flexible occlusive layer to the wound
    - waterproof and antibacterial
    - increases wound strength
    - also useful in emergency departments and primary care setting

Why do some grafts fail?

- Separation of graft from the underlying bed:
  - Shear
  - Haematoma
  - Infection
- Unsuitable bed (avascular)

Soft tissue sarcomas

How common are soft tissue sarcomas in adults?

- Account for 5–8% of all childhood cancers in European countries:
  - ◆ Nodular fasciitis (tender) a common differential diagnosis in young adults
- Most common sarcomas in childhood are:
  - ◆ *Rhabdomyosarcoma*: high metastatic potential
  - ◆ *Fibrosarcoma*: from birth onwards, metastatic potential depends on grade

How common are soft tissue sarcomas in adults?

- Comprise ~1% of all adult malignancies
- *Incidence*: 18 new cases per year per million population
- *Malignant fibrous histiocytoma (MFH)*: the most common in elderly men, mostly high grade and commonly lower limb
- *Leiomyosarcoma*: high distant metastasis rate, mainly in the skin, rarely deep seated
- *Liposarcoma*: patient in their 50s, larger tumours, lower extremity and low metastatic potential
- *Synovial sarcoma*: patients in their 30s, lower than upper extremeties, poor prognosis
- *Malignant peripheral nerve sheath tumour*: previously known as malignant schwannoma or neurofibrosarcoma
- *Angiosarcoma*: poor prognosis
- *Dermatofibrosarcoma protruberans (DFSP)*: well-differentiated fibrosarcoma, trunk, extremeties, head, early adult life and low metastatic potential
- *Epithelioid sarcoma*: commonly present as an ulcerating nodule hand or forearm
- *Retroperitoneal sarcomas*: account for 15% of all soft tissue sarcomas
  - ◆ 20% have lung mets at presentation
  - ◆ Liposarcomas account for over half

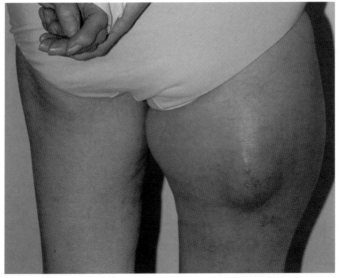

Soft tissue sarcoma of the right thigh in an 85 year old female at presentation to the Exeter Sarcoma Service.

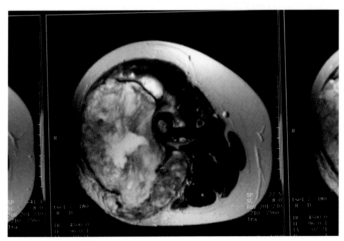

Magnetic resonance imaging confirms a massive tumour involving the lateral thigh.

Case Presentations in Plastic Surgery

What are the criteria for referral to a sarcoma unit?

- Any soft tissue mass >5 cm in size
- Any deep-seated mass
- Any rapidly increasing soft tissue mass
- Any painful mass

What determines the prognosis of a soft tissue sarcoma?

- Most sarcoma metastases are haematogenous (mostly to the lungs – 50% are solitary)
- Nodal spread can occur with synovial, epithelioid, clear cell and rhabdomyosarcoma
- Large, deep-seated and histologically high-grade lesions carry the worst prognosis
- Marginal resection leads to local recurrence but may not influence survival

How are soft tissue sarcomas managed?

- History and clinical examination
- Fine needle aspiration cytology (FNAC)
- Magnetic resonance imaging (MRI) scan with staging spiral computerised tomography (CT) scan of chest and abdomen
- Confirmatory core or open biopsy
- Definitive surgical resection
- Soft tissue reconstruction and limb preservation now preferred to limb amputation
- Neoadjuvant (in some high-grade tumours) or adjuvant chemotherapy or radiotherapy
- Pulmonary metastatectomy

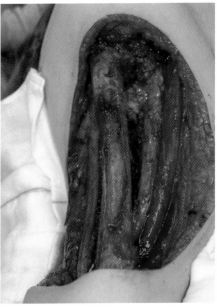

Large soft tissue defect created following limb-preserving resection of the tumour, viewed from laterally. From left to right can be seen the sciatic nerve, the femur (dissected subperiosteally over much of its length) and the superficial femoral vessels in the adductor canal, just deep to sartorius.

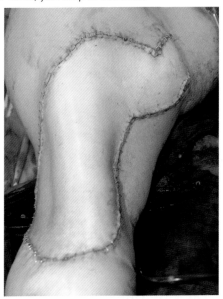

Soft tissue reconstruction achieved with an extended musculocutaneous 'pennant' flap pedicled on the deep inferior epigastric vessels with direct closure of the thoraco-abdominal donor site. This patient was ambulant at discharge at 2 weeks post-operatively with complete tumour clearance.

Case Presentations in Plastic Surgery

Squamous cell carcinoma

What is a squamous cell carcinoma (SCC)?

- A malignant epidermal tumour whose cells show maturation towards keratin formation

What factors have been implicated in the aetiology of SCC?

Ultra violet (UV) irradiation	Burn scar (Marjolin)
Osteomyelitis sinuses	Granulomatous infections
Hidradenitis supprativa	Dermatoses, such as poikiloderma
Venous ulcers	Industrial carcinogens and oils
Immunosuppression	Actinic keratoses and Bowen's disease
Xeroderma pigmentosa	Leucoplakia

Who is susceptible to developing SCC?

- Uncommon in dark-skinned races
- Late middle age onwards
- Male:female ratio 2:1

What are the clinical features of SCC?

- Firm skin tumour dorsum of hands, scalp and face
- Everted edges with a keratotic crust
- Well-differentiated tumours have a keratin horn
- Less-differentiated lesions flat and ulcerated

How is SCC treated?

- Excision with at least 5 mm margins where possible
- Monitor for lymph node or distant recurrence

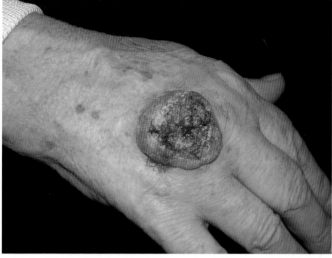

Typical appearance of a SCC on the dorsum of the hand.

Strawberry naevus (haemangioma)

What is a strawberry naevus?

- A benign neoplasm of vasoformative tissue (haemangioma)
- Well-defined life cycle of proliferation and involution
- 90% shortly after birth
- Grow rapidly in the first 5–8 months of life
- Regression: 50% aged 5 years, 60% aged 6 years, 70% aged 7 years, etc. to leave a pale pink scar

How can strawberry naevi be treated?

- Observation only
- Dressings for minor bleeding
- Corticosteroids: systemic or intralesional for the treatment of rapidly growing haemangiomas or those obstructing the airway or visual fields
- Surgery reserved for rapidly growing lesions unresponsive to medical treatment or where severe complications arise
- Uncomplicated haemangiomas should, in general, be left alone until complete involution

What are the potential complications associated with strawberry naevi?

- Ulceration, recurrent bleeding and infection
- Skeletal distortion
- High-output cardiac failure
- Late: scarring, residual colour mismatch, residual mass and redundant skin
- Kasabach–Merritt syndrome: sequestration of platelets leading to thrombocytopaenia, consumption coagulopathy and disseminated intravascular coagulation (DIC); leads to 30–40% mortality

Case Presentations in Plastic Surgery

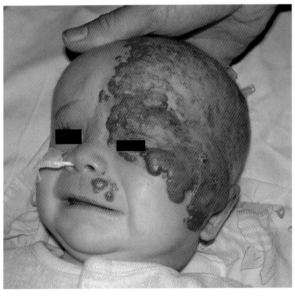

Large haemangioma affecting much of the face and scalp in an infant.

Syndactyly

How common is syndactyly (webbing) of the digits?

- Incidence 1 in 2000 live births
- May have a family history of syndactyly
- 50% bilaterality
- Twice as common in males
- The most affected web space is third, then fourth, second and first
- Commonly associated with almost any other congenital abnormality
- The second commonest congenital limb abnormality after polydactyly

How is syndactyly classified?

- Complete:
  - Digits united as far as distal phalanx
- Incomplete:
  - Syndactyly beyond mid-point of proximal phalanx but not to fingertips
- Complex:
  - Metacarpal or phalangeal synostosis (bone union)
- Simple:
  - No synostosis
- Acrosyndactyly:
  - Shortened digits united distally but with proximal fenestration
  - Association with constriction ring syndrome

When should surgery be undertaken?

- Most hand movements are learned between 6 and 24 months, so argument made for operating before 2 years of age
- Indications for early surgery in syndactyly:
  - Border digits
  - Length discrepancy

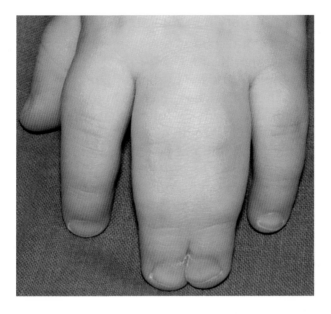

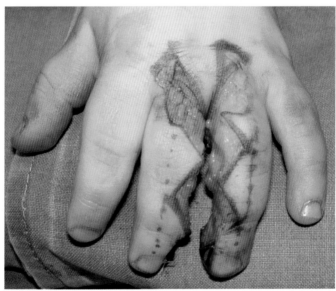

Complete, simple syndactyly affecting the middle and ring fingers before and after division. Skin grafts are used to reconstruct the skin deficit on each finger.

When should surgery be avoided?

- Minor degree of webbing, not cosmetically or functionally significant
- Severe complex syndactyly, digits share common structures including digital nerves and vessels
- Hypoplastic digits, where united digits function better than the two separated digits
- Adjacent webs should not be released simultaneously – risks vascularity
- Syndactyly of toes rarely corrected due to inevitable symptomatic hypertrophic scars

Tissue expansion

What is tissue expansion?

- The generation of new skin by the progressive expansion of a subcutaneous (s.c.) balloon via a remote or integral port
- Uses skin adjacent to a defect to enable replacement of like with like – colour, texture, hair-bearing quality and sensation
- Donor site can be closed directly

How is tissue expansion achieved?

- *Mechanical creep* is the elongation of skin under a constant load over time:
  - ◆ Collagen fibres stretch out and become parallel
  - ◆ Microfragmentation of elastin
- *Biological creep* is the generation of new tissue secondary to a persistent chronic stretching force (the type of creep seen in pregnancy)
- *Stress relaxation* describes the tendency for the resistance of the skin to a stretching force to decrease when held at a given tension over time
  - ◆ Skin is tight when just expanded, but in next visit skin is no longer tight

When is tissue expansion performed?

- Burn scar excision
- Alopecia (congenital and post-traumatic)
- Nasal reconstruction and ear reconstruction
- Excision of giant congenital naevi
- Excision of fasciotomy scars or skin grafted flap donor sites

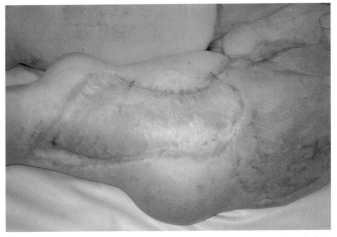

Tissue expanders have been inflated around the lateral thigh and medial knee prior to removal of mature skin graft on the anterior thigh. An expander in the medial thigh has already been removed due to exposure but has allowed for reduction of some of the grafted area at this site.

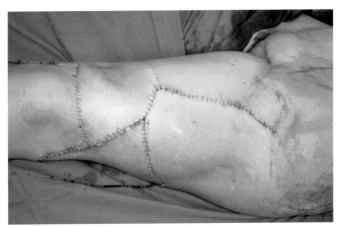

Following removal of the remaining expanders, the tissue generated has been used to reconstruct the anterior thigh with good quality skin.

What are the complications of tissue expansion?

- Extrusion
- Infection
- Rupture
- Wound dehiscence